An Introduction
to Epidemiologic Methods

Monographs in Epidemiology and Biostatistics
Edited by Abraham M. Lilienfeld

An Introduction
to Epidemiologic Methods

HAROLD A. KAHN

New York   Oxford
OXFORD UNIVERSITY PRESS
1983

Copyright © 1983 by Oxford University Press, Inc.

Library of Congress Cataloging in Publication Data
Kahn, Harold A.
  An introduction to epidemiologic methods.
  (Monographs in epidemiology and biostatistics; v. 5)
  Bibliography: p.   Includes index.
  1. Epidemiology—Methodology. I. Title. II. Series.
[DNLM: 1. Epidemiologic methods. WA 950 K12u]
RA652.4.K33   1983   614.4′072   82–14156

ISBN 0-19-503260-8
ISBN 0-19-503380-9 pbk.

Printing (last digit): 9 8 7 6 5 4 3 2 1

Printed in the United States of America

To the memory of my teachers
JEROME CORNFIELD
and
HAROLD F. DORN

Preface

This book is based on the author's experience in teaching a course on epidemiologic methods at the Johns Hopkins University School of Hygiene and Public Health. The students in this course are typically physicians, nurses, nutritionists, and other professionals who have become attracted to such fields as preventive medicine or public health and want to learn how to conduct an epidemiologic study or, as a minimum, how to appraise such a study conducted by others. With notable exceptions, these students are not well trained or skilled in quantitative methods. Thus the tone of this book is in accord with my experience that a deliberately detailed presentation emphasizing the sense of the matter and illustrating it with a numeric calculation is more successful than a cryptic outline, however rigorous. With regard to rigor, explanations herein are somewhat in keeping with the story about the student at Oxford who, when asked after an examination how he had proved the binomial theorem, replied cheerfully that, while he had not been able to prove the theorem, he had made it seem pretty plausible*. In some places I have attempted to include the bits and pieces that "everyone knows" . . . but many do not. To the extent that this makes reading the book too easy for some, I hope it is balanced by making it easy enough for others.

The prerequisites for Epidemiologic Methods at Hopkins are the basic course, Principles of Epidemiology, and at least one quarter of biostatistics. Although it is impossible to write a book on epidemiologic methods without reference to the principles of epidemiology, I have tried to do so. In more than a few instances the principles and the methods are so entwined that the reader of this book is given redundant instruction in basic principles. I do not apologize for this and believe it does no harm. Nonetheless, this work aims to

*J. R. Newman, *The World of Mathematics*. New York: Simon and Schuster, 1956.

be a book on methods and thus includes little or nothing on *why* one might prefer a retrospective or prospective study for a particular investigation or *why* one wishes to estimate an odds ratio or the probability of surviving, etc. To deal with these and related questions would require complete repetition of the basic course, and that I have not done.

With the very limited training in biostatistics required as a prerequisite, many students have to struggle to incorporate the concepts presented in the methods course into their existing framework of statistical ideas. This suggested to me the desirability of a review section, and so such a section has been included as Chapter 1.

Numeric examples that students can follow in detail have been included wherever practical, with emphasis placed on the approximate equality of numeric results obtained with different methods.

In summary, this book is based upon the viewpoint that, while all those involved in epidemiologic studies need to understand the fundamentals of data summarization and analysis, they need not become statisticians.

This book was written during my tenure as Lady Davis Visiting Professor of Epidemiology at the Hebrew University of Jerusalem. George Comstock, Sidney Cutler, Fred Ederer, Eric Peretz, Nathan Mantel, and James Schlesselman read the manuscript and offered helpful comments, suggestions, and criticisms that I wish to acknowledge with gratitude. My editor, Abraham Lilienfeld, merits a special thanks for his most generous assistance.

I am grateful to the literary executor of the late Sir Ronald A. Fisher, F. R. S.; to Frank Yates, F. R. S.; and to Longman Group, London, for permission to reprint random numbers from their book *Statistical Tables for Biological, Agricultural and Medical Research* (6th edn, 1974). I also wish to thank Jack Medalie and Uri Goldbourt for permission to use unpublished data from the Israeli Ischemic Heart Disease Study and Paolo Pasquini, Lawrence Gould, and Stanley Schor for permission to use unpublished data from the Merck Sharp and Dohme Research Laboratories.

Finally I wish to thank my wife, Lenora, for typing the manuscript and for support and encouragement in innumerable ways.

Loma Linda, California   H. A. K.
August 1982

Contents

An Introduction
to Epidemiologic Methods

1

Review of Selected
Elementary Statistics

Although almost all readers of this book will have completed one or more introductory statistics courses, my experience tells me that many students will benefit from a brief review of vocabulary, notation, elementary algebra, mean and variance formulas, and definition of chi-square. The items included in this review are needed to understand many of the epidemiologic methods to be discussed. This section is *not* a capsule review of an introductory statistics course and is not intended to be used as such.

VOCABULARY

A *population*, or *universe*, which should always be well defined by the investigator, can often be effectively described by certain summary constants called *parameters*. As an example we might cite the mean and standard deviation of systolic blood pressure values for all persons selected for service in the United States armed forces during the period 1942–1945. The complete set of blood pressure values for this group during 1942–1945 constitutes a population, and the mean and standard deviation of these values are parameters that, if known, can be used to describe this particular population. In this case, since the population values are almost certainly not normally distributed, the mean and standard deviation would not describe the population perfectly.

A random *sample* of blood pressure values could be taken from selective service records for 1942–1945 and the mean and standard deviation of the sample values calculated. These two summary values are called *statistics* and are generally used in estimating the corresponding *parameters*.

Systolic blood pressure is a variable reported in *discrete* values, such as 140, 126, 138. This variable is, however, at least in concept, a *continuous variable* and can assume any value within its range, such as 126.359021 . . . .

A special type of variable that we shall refer to frequently is the *attribute*. Attributes exist only in dichotomous form—sick or well, male or female, inducted into service or not inducted into service, etc.—and take on only the values 1 or 0.

A *null hypothesis* (H_0) states that the statistics (such as sample means) being compared are the result of random sampling from the same population and thus any difference between them is due to chance. A test of a null hypothesis is subject to two types of errors. *Type I error* is the result of rejecting the null hypothesis when it is in fact true. *Type II error* is the result of failing to reject the null hypothesis when it is in fact false. However, if the null hypothsis is true, type II error is nonexistent and irrelevant. Similarly, if the null hypothesis is false, type I error has no meaning. Because we do not know the actual facts of the populations from which our samples are derived (i.e., whether or not the null hypothesis is true), we invariably want studies that are designed to limit both types of errors. Thus *if* the null hypothesis is true, we want to limit the type I error to a value α, which is usually specified to be .01 or .05. If the null hypothesis is false and some alternative hypothesis (H_a) is true, we want to limit the type II error to a value β, commonly specified to be about .10. The *power* of a test to reject H_0 when H_a is true is equal to $1 - \beta$.

NOTATION AND ELEMENTARY ALGEBRA

The letters

$$X_1, X_2, \ldots, X_j, \ldots, X_N$$

represent values of a variable for the 1st, 2nd, $\ldots$, jth, $\ldots$, and Nth individuals in a *population* of size N.

The letters

$$x_1, x_2, \ldots, x_j, \ldots, x_n$$

represent values of a variable for the 1st, 2nd, $\ldots$, jth $\ldots$, and nth individuals in a *sample* of size n.

The notation

$$\sum_{j=1}^{N} X_j$$

represents the sum of all values of X_j from X_1 through and including X_N. Note: where the meaning is clear, we shall use $\sum X_j$ or even $\sum X$ to represent the sum of all values of X in place of the more complete notation.

The following are other common notations used in statistical analysis:

$|x|$ the absolute value of x, i.e., $|7|$ or $|-7| = 7$

$E(X)$ the expected value of X; equals each value of X multiplied by the

$\approx$ probability of that value, summed over all values; the mean value of X
        approximately equal to
$>$ greater than ($a > b$ indicates that a is greater than b)
$\geqslant$ greater than or equal to
$<$ less than ($a < b$ indicates that a is less than b)
$\leqslant$ less than or equal to

Note: students having difficulty remembering whether *less than* is represented by $<$ or by $>$ should note that the point of the wedge is next to the smaller quantity: $7 < 10$ and $5 > 2$.

If a quadratic equation is in the standard form

$$ax^2 + bx + c = 0$$

then

$$x = \frac{-b \pm \sqrt{b^2 - 4ac}}{2a}$$

If $10^x = y$, then x is the logarithm of y, using base 10.

If $e^x = y$, then x is the logarithm of y and y is the antilogarithm of x, both using base e.

The letter e represents the base used in natural logarithms and can be defined as the limiting value of the expression $(1 + \frac{1}{x})^x$ as x increases in size indefinitely. To illustrate: if $x = 2$, then $(1 + \frac{1}{2})^2 = (1.50)^2 = 2.250$; if $x = 100$, then $(1 + \frac{1}{100})^{100} = (1.01)^{100} = 2.705$. To three decimal places, $e = 2.718$. That is, even if $x = 1\,000\,000$ or more, $(1 + \frac{1}{x})^x$ will be less than 2.719. Hereafter, we shall refer only to logarithms using base e.

Also,

$\ln y = $ logarithm of y, using base e
$\ln (xy) = \ln x + \ln y$
$\ln (x/y) = \ln x - \ln y$
     $e^0 = e^{x-x} = e^x e^{-x} = 1$
     $e^{-x} = 1/e^x$
     $x^{1/2} = \sqrt{x}$

MEAN AND VARIANCE FORMULAS

The equations given below and the ideas corresponding to them occur frequently in epidemiologic analysis, and the reader should therefore be familiar with them.

$$\sum_{j=1}^{N} X_j/N = \mu \qquad\qquad (1\text{-}1)$$

where μ represents the mean of the population.

$$\sum_{j=1}^{N} (X_j - \mu)^2 / N = \text{var}(X) \qquad (1\text{-}2)$$

where var (X) represents the population variance.

$$\sum_{j=1}^{n} x_j / n = \bar{x} \qquad (1\text{-}3)$$

where $\bar{x}$ represents the mean of the sample. If the sample is picked at random, the expected value of $\bar{x}$, that is, its average value over all possible sample selections, is μ. In symbols,

$$E(\bar{x}) = \mu \qquad (1\text{-}4)$$

$$\sum_{j=1}^{n} (x_j - \bar{x})^2 / (n-1) = \hat{\text{var}}(X) \qquad (1\text{-}5)$$

where $\hat{\text{var}}(X)$ is an estimate of var (X) based on sample data. Note: when we are discussing both sample statistics and parameters or whenever necessary for clarity, we shall use a circumflex ($\hat{\ }$) to indicate the sample statistic and the absence of any such mark to indicate a parameter. Since parameters do not have variances, we can dispense with the circumflex over the statistic in expressions for the variance or the standard error of a statistic. We make two exceptions to these conventions. The first is for the parameter and statistic of a binomial distribution. Instead of P and $\hat{P}$ for the proportion with the characteristic under study, we shall use P and p for the *parameter* and *statistic*, respectively. The second exception is for the number of cases in each cell of a table. Here, too, the population values will be designated by capital letters—A, B, C, . . . —and the sample values by lower case letters—a, b, c, ...

$$\text{var}(\bar{x}) \cong \frac{\text{var}(X)}{n} \qquad \left(\text{unless } \frac{n}{N} > .10\right) \qquad (1\text{-}6)$$

$$\text{SE}(\bar{x}) \cong \left[\frac{\text{var}(X)}{n}\right]^{1/2} \qquad \left(\text{unless } \frac{n}{N} > .10\right) \qquad (1\text{-}7)$$

$\text{SE}(\bar{x})$ is the standard error of the sample mean. It is usually estimated by $\left[\dfrac{\hat{\text{var}}(X)}{n}\right]^{1/2}$, in which case we write $\hat{\text{SE}}(\bar{x})$. The variability of the sample mean, or any other sample statistic derived from a sample of size n, relates to the dispersion of an imaginary distribution of the sample statistic *in all possible samples* of size n from the population being sampled. The standard error of the sample statistic is, in fact, the standard deviation of this imaginary distribution.

VARIANCE FORMULAS FOR FUNCTIONS OF VARIABLES

The following formulas for the variance of simple functions are very useful.

$$\text{var}(X + Y) = \text{var}(X) + \text{var}(Y), \text{ if } X \text{ and } Y \text{ are independent} \qquad (1\text{-}8)$$

$$\text{var}(X - Y) = \text{var}(X) + \text{var}(Y), \text{ if } X \text{ and } Y \text{ are independent} \qquad (1\text{-}9)$$

$$\text{var}(KX) = K^2 \text{var}(X), \text{ where } K \text{ is a constant not subject to} \\ \text{sampling variation} \qquad (1\text{-}10)$$

MEAN AND VARIANCE FORMULAS FOR GROUPED DATA

Data are often summarized in groups, such as blood pressure classes 120–129, 130–139, ... The following definitions are used:

X_i = value assigned to each member of the ith class; usually taken as the midpoint of the ith class interval
f_i = number (frequency) of individuals in the ith class
m = number of classes

Then

$$\sum_{i=1}^{m} f_i X_i \bigg/ \sum_{i=1}^{m} f_i \cong \mu \qquad (1\text{-}11)$$

The approximation may be better or worse depending on the distribution of the actual values within each group.
Similarly,

$$\frac{\sum\limits_{i=1}^{m} f_i X_i^2}{\sum\limits_{i=1}^{m} f_i} - \left(\frac{\sum\limits_{i=1}^{m} f_i X_i}{\sum\limits_{i=1}^{m} f_i} \right)^2 \cong \text{var}(X) \qquad (1\text{-}12)$$

MEAN AND VARIANCE FORMULAS FOR ATTRIBUTE DATA

In a population where all values of X_i are either 1 or 0 (usually signifying the presence or absence of disease or some other attribute), let the proportion of the N values that are 1 be P. Then the frequency of 1's and 0's is NP and

$N(1 - P)$, respectively, and from Equations 1-11 and 1-12

$$\mu = \frac{NP(1) + N(1 - P)(0)}{NP + N(1 - P)} = P \tag{1-13}$$

$$\text{var}(X) = \frac{(NP)(1^2) + N(1 - P)(0^2)}{NP + N(1 - P)} - \left(\frac{NP(1) + N(1 - P)(0)}{NP + N(1 - P)}\right)^2$$

$$\text{var}(X) = \frac{NP}{N} - \left(\frac{NP}{N}\right)^2 = P - P^2 = P(1 - P) \tag{1-14}$$

In this case, the formulas for grouped data give exactly correct results because the two values are perfectly represented by the two X_i values. Thus P is the mean and $P(1 - P)$ is the variance of a population of 1's and 0's. If we take a sample of size n, the variance of the sample mean using Equation 1-6 is

$$\text{var}(\bar{x}) \cong \frac{\text{var}(X)}{n} = \frac{P(1 - P)}{n} \tag{1-15}$$

For attribute data, it is usual for p to be used in place of $\bar{x}$ for the sample mean, and thus we can write the above

$$\text{var}(p) \cong \frac{P(1 - P)}{n} \tag{1-16}$$

We rarely know P and usually estimate it with p. This leads to the usual formula

$$\hat{\text{var}}(p) \cong \frac{p(1 - p)}{n} \tag{1-17}$$

Sometimes, interest is focused not on the sample mean from an attribute population but on the number of 1's in the sample. In this case, the sample statistic to be considered is not p but np, which is the total number of individuals with the characteristic in the sample. Using Equation 1-17 for $\hat{\text{var}}(p)$ and Equation 1-10 on the variance of a variable multiplied by a constant, we have

$$\hat{\text{var}}(np) \cong \frac{n^2 p(1 - p)}{n} = np(1 - p) \tag{1-18}$$

It is very common for $(1 - P)$ and $(1 - p)$ to be written Q and q, respectively.

CONFIDENCE LIMITS

When a standard error of a sample mean has been calculated and the sample size is large or the population being sampled approximates a normal distribution, confidence limits (CL) for the population mean can be calculated as follows:

$$95\% \text{ CL} = \bar{x} \pm 1.96 \; \hat{SE}(\bar{x}) \qquad (1\text{-}19)$$

$$99\% \text{ CL} = \bar{x} \pm 2.58 \; \hat{SE}(\bar{x}) \qquad (1\text{-}20)$$

Note: as given, Equations 1-19 and 1-20 are not correct, even for large samples from a normal distribution. To make them exactly correct, we should substitute $SE(\bar{x})$ for $\hat{SE}(\bar{x})$. However, for large samples the distinction is slight. For small samples from a normal universe the values 1.96 and 2.58 should be changed in accordance with tables of Student's t values [1]. For small samples from a nonnormal universe, it may be advisable to consult with a statistician.

The justifications for using the confidence limits given above are that (a) the distribution of sample means in all possible samples from a normally distributed population is normal and (b) the distribution of all possible sample means based on large samples is approximately normal, whether or not the variable is normally distributed in the population being sampled. Our estimated standard error of the sample mean is an estimate of the standard deviation of the imaginary normal distribution of all possible sample means. In a normal distribution, only 5 percent of the values are more than ± 1.96 standard deviations away from the expected value. Since $E(\bar{x}) = \mu$, we can say that only 5 percent of the possible sample mean values are more than ± 1.96 $SE(\bar{x})$ distant from μ. We do not know $SE(\bar{x})$ but use instead $\hat{SE}(\bar{x})$, derived from sample data. For large samples, this is entirely satisfactory.

Assuming adequate sample size or normality of the population, we can add and subtract $1.96 \; \hat{SE}(\bar{x})$ to $\bar{x}$ and consider the resultant range to include μ. Only if our value of $\bar{x}$ is one of the 5 percent that are more than $\pm 1.96 \; \hat{SE}(\bar{x})$ distant from μ will our range of values fail to include μ. Thus $\bar{x} \pm 1.96 \; \hat{SE}(\bar{x})$ is a 95 percent confidence interval for μ. The identical argument applies to 99 percent confidence intervals using $\bar{x} \pm 2.58 \; \hat{SE}(\bar{x})$.

CHI-SQUARE FORMULAS

Most students of epidemiology are familiar with the formula relating χ^2 (chi square) to the quotient (observed frequency − expected frequency)^2 divided by expected frequency, summed over all the frequencies in a correlated set:

$$\chi^2 \equiv \sum \frac{(f_{obs} - f_{exp})^2}{f_{exp}}$$

Correlated frequencies are not all free to vary since if some observed frequencies are larger than expected, others will have to be smaller than expected. However, some students do not know that the above formula is a special instance of the basic formula for χ^2, which in the case of a single variable expressed as a deviation from its expected value is

$$\chi_1^2 = \frac{[x - E(x)]^2}{\text{var}(x)} \tag{1-21}$$

where the subscript 1 refers to one degree of freedom. In the case of K variables that are constrained to add to a fixed sum,

$$\chi_{(K-1)}^2 = \sum_{i=1}^{K} \frac{(x_i - \bar{x})^2}{\text{var}(x)} \tag{1-22}$$

2
Random Sampling

This book treats only samples that include a random element in the selection process. Nonrandom samples based on volunteers or on the judgment of the sampler as to the desirability or nondesirability of including a particular individual in the sample may be excellent or terrible as estimators of population parameters, but there is no objective way of judging which adjective applies. Statements such as "we are 95 percent confident that the mean percentage of cholesterol contained in high-density lipoproteins is between 17 and 19" can be made only for random samples.

SIMPLE RANDOM SAMPLING

Simple random sampling is simple in theory [2] but less so in practice. In theory, one has a list of N elements (usually individuals), a number is assigned in sequence from 1 to N to each element in sequence, and then a table of random numbers is used to select n individuals out of the N who are in the sample. For those unfamiliar with random number tables [3, 4, 5], a sample page of such a table is shown in Table 2-1 [6]. The mechanics of using the table are simple. Suppose, for example, that the population to be sampled has 8059 elements and a sample of 300 is to be selected. Consider the random number table in any arrangement that will produce a sequence of four-digit numbers. One way is to use columns of four digits. In Table 2-1, starting at the upper left corner of the page, this would result in 0347, 9774, 1676, etc. On reaching the bottom of the page, continue with the next column of four digits: 4373, 2467, etc. An alternative way of using the table is to select four-digit numbers from a single-digit vertical column. Using this procedure 0911, 5186, and 3512 would be the first three numbers in Table 2-1.

To avoid choosing the same sample each time, a method to vary the starting

Table 2-1. Random Sampling Numbers

03	47	43	73	86	36	96	47	36	61	46	98	63	71	62
97	74	24	67	62	42	81	14	57	20	42	53	32	37	32
16	76	62	27	66	56	50	26	71	07	32	90	79	78	53
12	56	85	99	26	96	96	68	27	31	05	03	72	93	15
55	59	56	35	64	38	54	82	46	22	31	62	43	09	90
16	22	77	94	39	49	54	43	54	82	17	37	93	23	78
84	42	17	53	31	57	24	55	06	88	77	04	74	47	67
63	01	63	78	59	16	95	55	67	19	98	10	50	71	75
33	21	12	34	29	78	64	56	07	82	52	42	07	44	38
57	60	86	32	44	09	47	27	96	54	49	17	46	09	62
18	18	07	92	46	44	17	16	58	09	79	83	86	19	62
26	62	38	97	75	84	16	07	44	99	83	11	46	32	24
23	42	40	64	74	82	97	77	77	81	07	45	32	14	08
52	36	28	19	95	50	92	26	11	97	00	56	76	31	38
37	85	94	35	12	83	39	50	08	30	42	34	07	96	88
70	29	17	12	13	40	33	20	38	26	13	89	51	03	74
56	62	18	37	35	96	83	50	87	75	97	12	25	93	47
99	49	57	22	77	88	42	95	45	72	16	64	36	16	00
16	08	15	04	72	33	27	14	34	09	45	59	34	68	49
31	16	93	32	43	50	27	89	87	19	20	15	37	00	49
68	34	30	13	70	55	74	30	77	40	44	22	78	84	26
74	57	25	65	76	59	29	97	68	60	71	91	38	67	54
27	42	37	86	53	48	55	90	65	72	96	57	69	36	10
00	39	68	29	61	66	37	32	20	30	77	84	57	03	29
29	94	98	94	24	68	49	69	10	82	53	75	91	93	30

Source: R. A. Fisher and F. Yates, *Statistical Tables for Biological, Agricultural, and Medical Research*. London: Longman, 1974 (by permission).

point is desirable. This method need not be elaborate. For example, perhaps opening a book to a "random" page shows pages 270 and 271. Use the first two digits of these pages as a starting point and begin with the twenty-seventh four-digit number in your random number table. In Table 2-1, using four-digit columns, this is 2467. Alternatively, the 27 could be used to begin with the seventh four-digit number on page 2 of the random number collection. Have some simple rule in mind and carry it through to produce a variable starting point. If more than one or two samples are to be selected, the method described below, while usable, is not the most efficient. The mechanics for allocation of a total population into K random samples, or subgroups, is described by Mantel [7].

We return now to the details of selecting 300 individuals from a population of 8059. In some way, perhaps using existing reference numbers (such as patients' clinic numbers or student identification card numbers), assign to each individual in the population one, and only one, four-digit number from 0001 to 8059. Using the numbers shown in Table 2-1 in the format of four-digit columns and using the twenty-seventh four-digit number as a starting point, the first ten random numbers are 2467, 6227, 8599, 5635, 7794, 1753, 6378, 1234, 8632, and 0792. Numbers 8599 and 8632 are not assigned to anyone in the population being sampled and thus have no relevance for this example of sample selection.

Thus, from the first ten random numbers, eight individuals are selected for the sample. Continue selecting individuals corresponding to the random numbers in the table until 300 sample individuals have been identified. This is the simple part of simple random sampling. The practical difficulties must now be confronted.

Nonresponse

If the study requires that a questionnaire be answered, will all 300 reply? If the study requires an examination, will all 300 submit to it? If the study requires merely abstracting information from existing records, is the specific information recorded for all 300? Perhaps the information is in the record but the record is missing from the file or otherwise unavailable. What is the importance of incomplete response and what can the investigator do about it?

Nonresponse is important because of the unknown differences between responders and nonresponders. The term *nonresponse* is used here in a general sense without regard to the specific reasons for nonresponse. One sample individual may refuse an examination. Another may be impossible to locate. In either case we should be concerned that those actually examined may differ in some important aspect from those not examined.

The problem of nonresponse is a general one. It applies to studies of total populations and of samples, to individuals lost from observation in longitudinal studies and to those not cooperative in cross-sectional studies. Writing specifically about incomplete follow-up, Lilienfeld and Lilienfeld state that differences between responders and nonresponders vary "in different studies and perhaps with different types of disease entities so that a general rule cannot be established . . ."[8].

The use of data derived from studies with moderate to large nonresponse rates usually presumes that the nonresponders are similar to those included, which may or may not be true. The investigator reporting sample data involving appreciable nonresponse has the burden of defending them and should supply supportive evidence with respect to the presumption of similarity. Dorn's comment on loss to follow-up can be generalized as, "The only correct way to deal with nonresponse is not to have any" [9]. There exists no certain method "not to have any," but the following guidelines may be useful.

1. Before embarking on any extensive study, conduct a pilot investigation, which among other benefits will provide some indication of the response rate. If it seems to be seriously low and cannot be improved, perhaps the study plan should be abandoned. If the study is to include long-term follow-up, a pilot investigation to test how many will stay under observation for ten years is clearly impractical. However, careful planning with respect to factors that may impair long-term follow-up can be helpful in defining the study population. A proposal to conduct a five-year study on the incidence of coronary disease among the Bedouin nomads of Israel was abandoned as soon as serious thought was given to the near impossibility of locating these wanderers some years after their initial examination.

2. Exert all practical effort toward obtaining cooperation from sampled individuals. A smaller sample intensively contacted with respect to cooperation may be preferable to a larger sample with a high nonresponse rate resulting from lack of resources to motivate cooperation.

3. If unable to obtain the cooperation of a sample individual with respect to the item under investigation, collect, where possible, such other information as may be helpful in judging whether or not the nonrespondent group differs in some respect from the respondents. A seroepidemiologic study of hepatitis B prevalence among recruits for military service in Italy included the collection of data on education, residence, etc., from all recruits, although 20 percent were rejected without being blood-tested. Comparison of those whose sera were tested with those whose sera were not tested with respect to the variables measured for both groups was helpful in calculating weighted estimates of the overall prevalence [10].

4. Intensive effort directed toward a subsample of the nonrespondent population is sometimes recommended and may help in estimating the extent of bias among nonrespondents. However, suppose n was the sample size considered appropriate for the study in order to measure a variable with adequate precision. Suppose that $n/3$ are nonrespondents and 25 percent of these ($n/12$) are intensively approached to obtain cooperation, with 100 percent success in the effort. The intensive effort will be costly, but since it applies to only one twelfth of the sample, it may be practical to carry out. This will result in $n/12$ individuals upon which to base estimates of the nonrespondents to see if they differ from the respondents. This, however, is $1/12$ the sample size believed necessary for adequate precision in measuring the variable of interest, as stated above. This approach is almost always helpful, but it is not a magic cure for the nonresponse problem.

The preceding discussion relates to moderate or large nonresponse rates. In this imperfect world, small nonresponse rates are necessarily acceptable. What then constitutes a response rate that is unacceptable or a cause for serious concern? There is no specific answer to that question in this book, or in any source that I am familiar with, and it is the investigator's responsibility to make a judgment as to the value of data based on a particular response rate.

The potential for bias is quite large in surveys of disease prevalence with high nonresponse rates. It is understandable that those with known disease may be uninterested, unable, or unwilling to respond. However, it is equally easy to appreciate that the sick may be specially interested in a study related to their condition and will therefore participate more readily than those who are well. Thus, good explanations exist for potential biases in opposite directions in the estimation of population prevalence of disease.

When the study objective is related to the association of two conditions, such as the development of myocardial infarction among those with and without high blood pressure, the likelihood of bias due to nonresponse seems less. Consider the population described by the simple cross-classification in Table 2-2. Two groups of persons who currently have high blood pressure are identified. The A group are those who will develop myocardial infarction in the next five years, and the B group are those who will not. At present, these two groups cannot be distinguished, and there is only the single group with high blood pressure, A + B. Estimates of the current prevalence of high blood pressure will be affected if the A + B group respond to the sample invitation to a greater or lesser extent than the group without high blood pressure, labeled C + D in Table 2-2. For the reasons previously cited, this is quite probable.

As shown in Table 2-3, however, even if the sample includes 10 percent of those with high blood pressure (A + B) and as many as 90 percent of those without high blood pressure (C + D), estimates of the degree of association of blood pressure with myocardial infarction incidence will still be almost unbiased, unless the 10 percent response for the A + B group is much greater than 10 percent for either the A or the B group and much less than 10 percent for the other. Similarly, if the 90 percent response in the C + D group differs greatly between C and D, bias will be introduced. While such variation cannot be ruled out, it is less likely than the differential participation of those currently sick relative to those currently well, as previously discussed.

Nonresponse has been discussed in this section on simple random sampling, but it is a matter of great concern to epidemiologists in many different types of

Table 2-2. Blood Pressure and Incidence of Myocardial Infarction in a *Population*

Present blood pressure	Will develop MI in next 5 years		
	Yes	No	Total
High	A	B	A + B
Normal	C	D	C + D

Odds ratio (Chapter 3) relating MI and blood pressure level in population = AD/BC.

Table 2-3. Blood Pressure and Incidence of Myocardial Infarction in a *Sample*

Present blood pressure	Will develop MI in next 5 years		
	Yes	No	Total
High	$\dfrac{A^a}{10}$	$\dfrac{B}{10}$	$\dfrac{A+B}{10}$
Normal	$\dfrac{9C}{10}$	$\dfrac{9D}{10}$	$\dfrac{9(C+D)}{10}$

Odds ratio (Chapter 3) relating MI and blood pressure level in sample $= (A/10)(9D/10) \div (B/10)(9C/10) = [AD(9)/100][100/BC(9)] = AD/BC$, as in Table 2-2 for the population.

[a] Ten percent of high blood pressure population and 90 % of normal blood pressure population are in the sample.

investigations. It is an ever-present concern with regard to any type of sampling, and even if a complete population is being followed, failure to remain under observation is equivalent to nonresponse for a portion of the study. When studying epidemiologic data of any kind, it is always worthwhile to consider if the included individuals fairly represent the population under study. The extent of nonresponse is an important element in this appraisal.

STRATIFIED RANDOM SAMPLING

Sometimes it is possible to identify separate sections of the population, which we call *strata*, and to take advantage of them in our sampling plan so as to reduce the sampling error below that for a simple random sample. The fundamental aspect of stratified sampling is that the strata are sampled separately and the results then appropriately combined in the analysis. If much of the variability in what we are measuring is between strata, we can use stratification to reduce sampling variance. By sampling within strata and then combining the results appropriately, our results are completely free of the variability between strata, however great that might be.

An extreme (unrealistic) example illustrates this idea. A sample study is proposed to estimate the average length of postoperative hospital stay for a certain disease. Separate lists exist (or information is available that allows us to make such lists) for hospitals having fewer than 25 beds, those having 25 to 99 beds, and those having 100 beds or more. Suppose further that all hospitals with fewer than 25 beds keep such patients exactly nine days, all hospitals of 25 to 99 beds keep such patients exactly seven days, and hospitals of 100 beds or larger keep these patients exactly five days. By simple sampling of a combined list that includes all sizes of hospitals, it would be possible to get samples with averages as low as five days and as high as nine days. With stratified sampling, however, the estimate for hospitals with fewer than 25 beds would always be nine days, no matter which hospitals of this group were selected. Similarly, the possible samples for the other strata could yield only the sample means of five days and seven days, regardless of which hospitals were selected within each stratum. In this extreme case, all of the variance in length of stay is between strata. *Within each stratum* there is no variance at all. Using stratified sampling (and suitable combination of the results of each stratum's sample into an overall average), there would be no sampling variance. All possible samples would yield the same results.

One other artificial example illustrates the potential benefits of stratification. Imagine a population, or universe, consisting of just eight elements as follows: 0_a 0_b 0_c 0_d 1_a 1_b 1_c 1_d, with subscripts used to permit identification of individual elements. Our purpose in introducing this miniuniverse is to permit students to hold in their hand, so to speak, some of the elements of sampling theory. For any real example, we can only appeal to concepts, but through the device of this miniuniverse, students can get a feel for what is meant by "all possible samples," "standard error of the mean," etc. The superficial point of the illustration is to show how sample design (simple or stratified random) affects sampling variance. The deeper purpose is to give students clearer insight into the fundamentals of sampling theory without the necessity of working through that theory.

For this population, $P = 0.5$ is the mean and $P(1 - P) = 0.25$ is the variance. A simple sample of size 2 might result in any one of the 28 possible samples listed in Table 2-4. Summarizing these and ignoring the individual identification, we get:

Sample	Sample Mean	Frequency
0–0	0	6
0–1	0.5	16
1–1	1.0	6
All		28*

Table 2-4. All Possible Samples of Size 2 in Simple Random Sampling from a Population Consisting of $0_a0_b0_c0_d1_a1_b1_c1_d$

0_a0_b	0_b0_c	0_c1_a	0_d1_d
0_a0_c	0_b0_d	0_c1_b	1_a1_b
0_a0_d	0_b1_a	0_c1_c	1_a1_c
0_a1_a	0_b1_b	0_c1_d	1_a1_d
0_a1_b	0_b1_c	0_d1_a	1_b1_c
0_a1_c	0_b1_d	0_d1_b	1_b1_d
0_a1_d	0_c0_d	0_d1_c	1_c1_d

To calculate the mean and variance of this distribution of all possible sample means of size 2, we use Equations 1-11 and 1-12 on the following data:

$\bar{x}$	f	$f\bar{x}$	$f\bar{x}^2$
0	6	0	0
0.5	16	8.0	4.0
1.0	6	6.0	6.0
	28	14.0	10.0

The mean of all possible sample means is

$$\frac{\sum f\bar{x}}{\sum f} = \frac{14}{28} = 0.5 = P$$

Note that the mean of all possible sample means equals P, the mean of the universe from which we are sampling. Thus, our sample means are unbiased estimates of the population mean. The standard error of the sample mean is the standard deviation of the *distribution of all possible sample means*, which equals

$$\left[\frac{\sum f\bar{x}^2}{\sum f} - \left(\frac{\sum f\bar{x}}{\sum f}\right)^2\right]^{1/2} = \left[\frac{10.0}{28.0} - (0.5)^2\right]^{1/2} = \left(\frac{3}{28}\right)^{1/2}$$

In real sampling applications, the number of all possible samples becomes enormous and the distribution of all possible sample means is only a concept and not an actual enumerated distribution. In the example cited earlier of a sample of 300 from a population of 8059, there are over 10^{554} different samples possible. Obviously, the standard error of the sample mean applicable to real samples needs to be determined by methods other than the direct calculation of the standard deviation of all possible means. It is, of course, calculated by formula. The formula for simple sampling appropriate for either binomial or continuous variables is

$$[\text{var}(\bar{x})]^{1/2} = \left[\frac{\text{var}(X)}{n}\left(\frac{N-n}{N-1}\right)\right]^{1/2} \tag{2-1}$$

the term $(N-n)/(N-1)$, called the *finite sampling factor*, is useful whenever the sample represents 10 percent or more of the total population; otherwise it may be omitted. Equation 1-6 for the variance of a sample mean and Equation 1-7 for the standard error of a sample mean did not include the finite sampling factor and thus were shown as approximations that would be satisfactory unless $(n/N) > .10$.

In practical sampling problems, $\text{var}(X)$ is usually unknown and $\hat{\text{var}}(X)$ is used as an estimate. In the artificial example we are investigating, $\text{var}(X)$ is known and its use in Equation 2-1 results in

$$[\text{var}(\bar{x})]^{1/2} = \left[\frac{.5(.5)}{2}\left(\frac{8-2}{8-1}\right)\right]^{1/2} = \left[\frac{1}{8}\left(\frac{6}{7}\right)\right]^{1/2} = \left(\frac{3}{28}\right)^{1/2}$$

exactly as calculated by direct enumeration.

If by the use of supplementary information, such as sex, area, or age, for example, we were able to divide the population into two strata that tended to include the 1's in one stratum and the 0's in the other, we might have

$$\text{Stratum 1} \qquad 0_d 1_a 1_b 1_c$$

$$\text{Stratum 2} \qquad 1_d 0_a 0_b 0_c$$

We can now select a stratified sample of size 2 by taking one element at random from stratum 1 and one element at random from stratum 2. Under these conditions the possible sample selections are

From Stratum 1	From Stratum 2
0_d	1_d
0_d	0_a
0_d	0_b
0_d	0_c
1_a	1_d
1_a	0_a
1_a	0_b
1_a	0_c
1_b	1_d
1_b	0_a
1_b	0_b
1_b	0_c
1_c	1_d
1_c	0_a
1_c	0_b
1_c	0_c

Combining samples of similar composition by ignoring identification of individual elements results in

Sample	Sample Mean	Frequency
0–0	0	3
0–1	0.5	10
1–1	1.0	3
All		16†

The reduction in total number of possible samples from 28 to 16 is characteristic of stratified sampling. This can easily be understood by recognizing that some of the samples possible under simple sampling are no longer possible when a stratified sampling procedure is used. For example, selection of 1_a and 1_b from stratum 1 is not possible under the stratified plan of selecting one from each stratum; however, the combination of 1_a and 1_b is one of the possibilities in simple sampling.

We now calculate the mean and variance of the 16 possible sample means of size 2 from the stratified sample:

$\bar{x}$	f	$f\bar{x}$	$f\bar{x}^2$
0	3	0	0
0.5	10	5.0	2.50
1.0	3	3.0	3.00
	16	8.0	5.50

The mean of all possible sample means is

$$\frac{\sum f\bar{x}}{\sum f} = \frac{8.0}{16.0} = 0.5 = P$$

In this illustration of stratified sampling, our results show that the mean of all possible sample means is the mean of the universe. When this is the case, the sample mean is said to be *unbiased*.

The variance of all possible sample means is

$$\frac{\sum f\bar{x}^2}{\sum f} - \left(\frac{\sum f\bar{x}}{\sum f}\right)^2 = \frac{5.50}{16} - (0.5)^2 = \frac{3}{32}$$

and the standard deviation of all possible sample means is $\left(\frac{3}{32}\right)^{1/2}$. Equation 2-2 is appropriate for estimating the overall population mean using data from a stratified sample:

$$\bar{x}(\text{strat}) = \sum_{i=1}^{r} \frac{N_i}{N} \bar{x}_i \qquad (2\text{-}2)$$

where $\bar{x}_i$ is the sample mean of the ith stratum and r equals the number of strata $(i = 1, 2, \ldots, r)$.

Weighting the sample mean of the ith stratum $(\bar{x}_i)$ by the proportion that the ith stratum size is of the total population size provides an unbiased estimate of the overall mean. Note that the weighting factors relate to population sizes (N_i and N) and not to sample sizes (n_i and n). If stratified sampling allocation of n_i is not proportional to stratum sizes, n_i/n will differ from N_i/N, and it is N_i/N

that is the proper weighting factor. The variance of an overall stratified sample mean derived by weighting the sample means for individual strata as in Equation 2-2 is

$$\text{var}(\bar{x}) \text{ strat} = \sum_{i=1}^{r} \left(\frac{N_i}{N}\right)^2 \frac{\text{var}_i(x)}{n_i} \left(\frac{N_i - n_i}{N_i - 1}\right) \tag{2-3}$$

where $\text{var}_i(x)$ is the variance of x within the ith stratum.

Applying Equation 2-3 to our artificial example of sample size 2, we obtain

$$\text{var}(\bar{x}) \text{ strat} = \left(\frac{4}{8}\right)^2 \frac{.75\,(.25)}{1} \left(\frac{4-1}{4-1}\right) + \left(\frac{4}{8}\right)^2 \frac{.25\,(.75)}{1} \left(\frac{4-1}{4-1}\right)$$

$$= \frac{1}{4}\left(\frac{3}{4}\right)\left(\frac{1}{4}\right) + \frac{1}{4}\left(\frac{1}{4}\right)\left(\frac{3}{4}\right) = \frac{6}{64} = \frac{3}{32}$$

as the variance of the distribution of all possible stratified means of size 2. The square root of this, $(3/32)^{1/2}$, is the standard deviation of this distribution and is the standard error of $\bar{x}$ (strat). The value $(3/32)^{1/2}$ is exactly equal to what we obtained earlier as the standard deviation of all possible stratified samples of size 2.

Recalling that the standard error of $\bar{x}$ (simple) was $(3/28)^{1/2}$, we see, in this artificial example, that stratification may result in reduction of sampling error. If the allocation of sample n_i to the several strata is proportional to stratum size (N_i), then the variance of $\bar{x}$ (strat) will be the same as or less than the variance of $\bar{x}$ (simple) for samples of the same size. The reduced variance for stratified sampling depends on the differences between strata for the variable of interest. The more stratum means differ from each other, and the more strata are alike within themselves, i.e., the smaller the variance within strata, the more potential benefit there is in stratified sampling.

If the investigator has a reasonably good basis for estimating $[\text{var}(x)]^{1/2}$—for the binomial this is equivalent to estimating P_i since $(P_i Q_i)^{1/2} = [\text{var}(x)]^{1/2}$—for the several strata and believes they differ appreciably, consideration should be given to allocating n_i proportional to

$$\frac{N_i[\text{var}_i(x)]^{1/2}}{\sum_i N_i[\text{var}_i(x)]^{1/2}}$$

This is called *optimum allocation* and provides the smallest possible sampling variance obtainable with stratified sampling, provided the estimates of $[\text{var}_i(x)]^{1/2}$ are not far from the truth. Although sample size in each stratum may be determined by optimum allocation as just described, by proportional allocation, or otherwise, Equation 2-2 provides the correct estimate of the overall mean. If optimum allocation is attempted on the basis of poor estimates of $[\text{var}_i(x)]^{1/2}$, it is possible that the resultant sampling variance will be larger than for simple random sampling.

To summarize, allocate stratified sample size proportional to N_i unless you have good reason to do otherwise.

Do not forget that all of the practical problems concerning nonresponse discussed under simple sampling apply to stratified sampling and to every other type of sampling as well.

SYSTEMATIC SAMPLING

Systematic sampling is a common type of sampling based on selecting every rth individual from a list or file after choosing a random number from 1 to r as a starting point. Going back to the example used for simple random sampling, choosing 300 from a population of 8059, we now obtain a systematic sample by calculating the ratio $8059/300 = 26.9$ and selecting every twenty-sixth (or twenty-seventh) individual in the file after a random start between 1 and 26 (or 27). Note that using $r = 26$ results in a sample size of 309 and $r = 27$ results in a sample size of 298. It is typical of systematic sampling procedures that they yield sample sizes approximately, rather than exactly, equal to the targeted sample size.

Systematic sampling is based on a fixed nonrandom rule and is not limited to selection from an actual file. Thus, selection of all those born on the (randomly chosen) fifth day of any month or of everyone whose social security number ends in (the randomly chosen digits) 12, 65, or 87 is similar to systematic sampling procedures yielding approximately 3 percent samples. Of course, the choice of the sampling scheme has to be relevant to the population being sampled. A population that is not completely covered by social security would be unsuitable for sampling by means of social security numbers. A primitive population that did not record and remember birthdays could not be sampled using date of birth.

The reason for the popularity of systematic sampling is its simplicity and, in many instances, its superiority over simple sampling. The simplicity is obvious, the potential superiority less so. We shall consider this aspect in terms of an example. Suppose we want to systematically sample a chronological list of all hospital admissions for one year. If the sampling objective is to estimate the proportion of all hospital admissions during the year that are due to infectious diseases, it is quite probable that a systematic sample of admissions is preferable to a simple random sample. Consider that admissions for infectious diseases may have seasonal peaks and that by systematic sampling from a chronological list we are sure to obtain $(1/r)$th of the admissions in each season. In simple random sampling, however, some of the possible samples would include admissions only from a particular season and thereby improperly reflect the proportion of annual admissions for infectious disease. As in the foregoing example, if the list is ordered in a manner related to the study objective, systematic sampling is in some respects analogous to stratified sampling. If the list is in random order, systematic sampling is analogous to simple random sampling.

If however, the list is in cyclical order so that every rth element is in some way special, then systematic sampling can be disastrous. Investigators must be on guard with regard to this last situation, but it rarely occurs. An example commonly cited relates to choosing a sample of homes. In such a situation, it is possible that if the random start provides a corner house, every rth house thereafter might also be a corner house. If corner houses are related to above-average economic status or above-average family size or some other aspect of relevance to the study, systematic sampling might provide misleading data. As stated earlier, such a constellation of events is not very probable, but be sure to give it some thought.

How should the sampling variance of means derived from systematic sampling be estimated? Whereas the number of possible simple random samples of 300 from 8059 is more than 10^{554}, the number of possible samples of 309 using systematic sampling from a list of 8059 is *only* 26. There are 26 possible starting points on the list in accordance with the random number chosen and thus only 26 possible different systematic samples. Clearly the distribution of all possible sample means and consequently the formulas for calculating the sampling error for simple samples (and also within strata for stratified samples) do not apply to systematic sampling. There are formulas that depend on the serial correlation coefficient [11] and split sample methods, but they are clumsy to apply [12]. However, my recommendation is to use Equation 1-6 for simple random sampling and to consider the results as approximately correct if the list being used is ordered at random or not ordered in any way known to be relevant to the variable of interest. The formulas applicable to simple random sampling can be considered as overstating the sampling variability if the ordering of the list is relevant to the variable under study.

For systematic samples not derived from a real list, such as the example given of choosing all those born on the fifth of any month, we must first be able to assume that the day of the month is unrelated to our study objectives. Without this qualification, we would not have a random element in our sample. Next, we must recognize that such a sample, which in this case is made up of all those born on the fifth of the month, lacks the characteristics of a systematic sample drawn from a list whose order is in some way relevant to study interests. We have no guarantee that using birth date we will get about one thirtieth of those of every age, one thirtieth of those living in every geographic section, one thirtieth of the men, one thirtieth of the women, etc., but instead we have an excellent approximation to the size and kind of sample we would have obtained by sampling every thirtieth from a list arranged at random.

The selection of every rth person from a list ordered by age is an excellent approximation to stratified sampling with proportional allocation. If the list ordering is relevant to what we want to measure—and age is relevant to practically everything the epidemiologist is interested in measuring—the sections of the list may be thought of as strata that differ as to strata means. This is the feature of list ordering that provides the basis for reduction in sampling variance.

The increased efficiency of systematic sampling can be substantial, but it is altogether dependent on the degree to which the variable of interest is associated with the order of population elements on the list. Although systematic sampling can be equivalent to a type of stratified sampling, there is no practical way to use the standard error formulas appropriate to stratified sampling.

CLUSTER SAMPLING

The individuals in the population we wish to sample are often grouped into clusters, e.g., families, villages, or hospital wards. Although it is often convenient or administratively desirable to first sample clusters and then investigate the individuals in the chosen clusters rather than to sample individuals directly from the population, the effect on sample results needs to be understood. There is an important distinction, for example, between picking a sample of 1000 from a population of 100 000 by direct random selection and picking 1000 individuals from 250 randomly selected nuclear families.

To illustrate the problem, we consider estimating the proportion of 1981 hospitalized patients diagnosed as having myocardial infarction who report having taken a specified amount, or more, of aspirin during the week prior to diagnosis. Depending upon study objectives, the investigator may wish to compare the proportion of myocardial infarction patients positive for aspirin with suitable controls. However, for the purpose of discussing and explaining cluster sampling, reference to the hospitalized patients only will be sufficient.

Assume that, in the study area, there are 17 hospitals treating myocardial infarction patients, that during 1981 they discharged about 1000 such patients, and that we need about 250 cases for the precision desired. Further assume that the hospitals are generally similar with respect to patient populations, accuracy in diagnosis, etc.

We might, of course, proceed by simple random, stratified random, or systematic random methods to select 250 of the 1000 patients for inclusion in the study. However, to carry out such a study we would have to assign a part-time interviewer to each hospital and the expense would be much greater than if the study could be limited to a few hospitals. Each hospital represents a cluster of patients, and to use cluster sampling, we first pick several hospitals at random. In the present example, perhaps 6 of the 17 would be selected and then only the MI patients or a sample of the MI patients in these six hospitals would be included in the study.

The greater ease and convenience of carrying out a study in 6 rather than 17 hospitals is evident. What then is the drawback? Why are not all sample studies initiated by selection of convenient clusters? The answer to both questions is that sampling variance is likely to be increased. Although likely, it is not a certainty that cluster sampling variance will be larger than simple random sampling variance, and there is even some chance that cluster sampling variance will be smaller.

We use an extreme example to explain how selecting clusters affects sampling variance. Suppose a population consists of three clusters, A, B, and C. For the variable of interest, each cluster is composed of perfectly homogenous elements, i.e., every individual in a cluster is like every other individual in that cluster. Assume that our variable is the presence of rheumatoid arthritis and that each cluster is made up of only one type of individual. In cluster A all are negative, in cluster B all are positive, and in cluster C all are doubtful with respect to rheumatoid arthritis. We now pick one cluster at random and then study all or a sample of all the individuals therein with respect to rheumatoid arthritis. No matter how large our sample size is, it is clear that we cannot learn anything more about the cluster than could have been learned by a sample of one from the same cluster. Furthermore, we have no indication that the individuals in the two clusters not selected are completely different from the individuals in our sample. Of course, this is an extreme example, but it illustrates the fact that if the characteristic of interest is positively correlated within clusters, as is very often the case ("birds of a feather flock together"), n sample observations will produce fewer than n independent units of information. In addition, if clusters vary greatly from one to another so that at least some of them must deviate substantially from population parameters, the clusters selected may not provide good estimates of the proportion of the total population having the characteristic being studied.

If clusters are random assemblages of individuals, then cluster sampling has no greater sampling variance than simple random sampling. In this case it is wise to take advantage of the practical benefits of cluster sampling. However, if clusters are positively correlated within themselves, i.e., more homogenity than would result from chance association, cluster sampling variance will be larger than simple random sampling variance. If clusters are negatively correlated within themselves, however, i.e., more heterogeneity than would result from chance association, cluster sampling benefits the investigator both by reduced variance for fixed sample size and by reduced costs. Since calculation of cluster sampling variance depends on the intraclass correlation coefficient [12], which epidemiologists are unlikely to know, my advice is the converse of that for systematic sampling. Estimate the variance of cluster sampling by using the formula for simple random sampling (Equation 1-6) but recognize that, in practically all instances, this will be an underestimate of true variance. Only if clusters are formed at random or reflect negative correlation within themselves for the variable of interest will the variance obtained from the simple random sampling formula equal or overestimate the real sampling variance of cluster sampling.

SAMPLE SIZE

"How large a sample do I need?" is a frequent question, and we shall first consider it from the viewpoint of simple random sampling and then indicate how sample size is affected by stratified, systematic, and cluser sampling methods.

We consider three types of sample size calculations and, for ease of exposition, initially limit our consideration to binomial variables. First and simplest is the sample size needed to estimate a single binomial parameter with a specified precision. Suppose we wish to estimate the proportion of regular current cigarette smokers in the freshman class entering a large university and we would like our estimate to have a high probability of being within $\pm \Delta$ of the true value, where Δ signifies a specific difference (such as .03 or .05) between our estimate and the true value.

Before calculating the sample size needed in order to estimate the proportion of freshmen who smoke cigarettes, we must take what seems to be a ridiculous step: we must estimate what that proportion is. The basic reason for this is that sample size depends on the standard error of the variable to be estimated, and, as was shown earlier, the standard error of p equals

$$\left[\frac{P(1-P)}{n}\right]^{1/2}$$

Suppose we judge the proportion of cigarette smoking among freshmen to be .30 and specify Δ as .04; then

$$1.96 \ \mathrm{SE}(p) = 1.96\left[\frac{P(1-P)}{n}\right]^{1/2} = .04 \qquad (2\text{-}4)$$

$$= 1.96\left[\frac{(.30)(.70)}{n}\right]^{1/2} = .04$$

expresses the prior opinion that we would like 1.96 standard errors of our estimate to equal .04. If $1.96 \ \mathrm{SE}(p) = .04$, then our sample estimate has about a 95 percent chance of being within four percentage points of the truth. This assumes that n is large enough to make the distribution of all possible sample p values approximately normal. For epidemiologic studies this is usually the case. We can now solve for n. Doing this, we get $n = 504$. Thus if the true value is in fact .30, the mean of a sample of size 504 will be within $\pm$ .04 of .30, or from .26 to .34, 95 percent of the time. We now repeat these calculations assuming $P = .10, .20, .40,$ and .50:

$$1.96\left[\frac{(.10)(.90)}{n}\right]^{1/2} = .04 \qquad n = 216$$

$$1.96\left[\frac{(.20)(.80)}{n}\right]^{1/2} = .04 \qquad n = 384$$

$$1.96\left[\frac{(.40)(.60)}{n}\right]^{1/2} = .04 \qquad n = 576$$

$$1.96\left[\frac{(.50)(.50)}{n}\right]^{1/2} = .04 \qquad n = 600$$

Table 2-5. Sample Size Required for Selected Values
of P with .95 Confidence Limits Fixed at ± .04

P	Sample size	95 % of sample p's will be between
.10	216	.06 and .14
.20	384	.16 and .24
.30	504	.26 and .34
.40	576	.36 and .44
.50	600	.46 and .54

The corresponding ranges within which 95 percent of sample p values fall are
given in Table 2-5.

What happens if our estimate of P is a poor one? Suppose we estimate
$P = .20$ and calculate a sample size of 384, but in fact P is .40. With $P = .40$, the
true variance of all possible sample means of size 384 is $(.4)(.6)/384 = .000625$,
with standard error of the sample mean equal to $(.000625)^{1/2}$, or .025. Two
standard errors would equal .05, and 95 percent of the sample p's based on a
sample size of 384 would be between .35 and .45. If we observe a p of .35 in our
sample and use it to estimate SE(p), we would estimate the true mean as
between .30 and .40 with .95 confidence. Of course, we are going to take not all
possible samples but only one, and it may happen that the p for the sample we
select is extremely low. In that case we might continue to think that the true
value is about .20. However, it is much more likely that the sample result will
contribute to changing our prior opinion about the prevalence of cigarette
smoking among freshmen.

This illustration of results following a poor estimate of P indicates that
useful findings may not be critically dependent on good preliminary estimates
of P.

Let us examine this same question of the sample size needed to estimate a
single parameter with a specified precision from a slightly different viewpoint.
Suppose instead of specifying precision as within four percentage points, we
specify precision as a proportion of P. If we want 1.96 SE(p) to equal $P/5$, this
would be equivalent to $\pm .05$ if $P = .25$ and to $\pm .02$ if $P = .10$. Often this is the
better way to describe desired accuracy. For example, the specification $\pm .05$ is
not too useful if $P = .01$. To set up the equation in this form, with
1.96 SE $(p) = P/K$, we have

$$1.96 \ SE(p) = 1.96 \left[\frac{P(1-P)}{n} \right]^{1/2} = \frac{P}{K} \qquad (2\text{-}5)$$

If K is specified as 5, we need only insert our preliminary estimate of P and then
solve for n.

For $P = .01$, the specification that 95 percent of samples should fall between
.008 and .012 requires an n of 9508. This rather large sample size could exceed

the total size of the freshmen class, which would certainly remind us to use the finite sampling factor, $[(N - n)/(N - 1)]$, as part of the variance equation. If the total freshmen class at our hypothetical large university were 5000, the equation to solve for n with $P = .01$ and approximately 95 percent assurance of $\pm P/5$ is

$$1.96 \left[\frac{.01(.99)}{n} \left(\frac{N - n}{N} \right) \right]^{1/2} = \frac{.01}{5} \qquad n \cong 3300$$

Note that to simplify the arithmetic we use N instead of $N - 1$ in the denominator of the finite sampling factor. For $N = 5000$, this is an inconsequential change.

Comparision of Two Groups

Often the epidemiologist's interest is not in estimating a single parameter but in comparing two parameters. The sample size needed for a randomized, controlled clinical trial is an example. Suppose it is proposed to conduct a trial of some type of medication or diet to study its effect on reducing the incidence of myocardial infarction. Setting aside the many practical problems of conducting such a trial [13], we direct our attention to estimating the sample size needed.

In order to estimate the sample size needed for a study capable of detecting a change in incidence rate, it is necessary to have a preliminary estimate of what that incidence rate is. Suppose we are planning a three-year study and have data suggesting that the population we intend to study, taking into account age, sex, etc., has an incidence rate of new cases of myocardial infarction of 1 percent per year, or about 3 percent for the three-year study period. In addition to estimating the existing incidence rate, it is necessary to stipulate what degree of change (associated with the treatment being investigated) the study is supposed to detect with a high probability. The difference to be detected (i.e., if it exists, we shall have a high probability of not missing it) is determined by a blend of subject matter considerations and the investigator's judgment. Determining whether a proposed program might reduce the annual incidence of myocardial infarction from .030 to .029 seems inappropriate. Conceivably circumstances may exist in which detection of this change is desirable, but in general it is unwise to try and identify such a small difference. A program causing a slight reduction is very likely to be superseded before long by some improved alternative. Thus a difficult, expensive, and time-consuming study might come to the conclusion that program A does seem to reduce annual incidence by .001, only to be overtaken by the emergence of program B, which is thought to lower incidence by .005.

If the true control group incidence rate is 3 percent per three-year study period and the treatment reduces this to 2.9 percent, the sample size needed to detect this slight difference will necessarily be larger than the sample size needed to detect a reduction from 3 percent to 1 percent. In general, the larger the difference to be detected, the smaller the sample size required. (Using the word *detect* is a form of shorthand because what we are actually referring to is the detection of a statistically significant difference between the two groups.) If the control and treatment incidence rates are as stipulated, the four factors we must know for calculating the sample size needed in order to have a stated probability of detecting a significant difference are

P_c true incidence rate in the control group
P_e true incidence rate in the experimental group
α probability of type I error in performing the test of significance, i.e., concluding that there is a difference between P_c and P_e when in fact the sample data regarding each are only random variations arising from the same parameter, P_c
β probability of type II error in performing the test of significance, i.e., failing to reject the null hypothesis when in fact P_c and P_e differ *as stipulated*

Before putting these components together in a way that will enable the various formulas for sample size calculation to make sense, I remind readers about the variance of the difference between *independent variables* as previously stated in Equation 1-9:

$$\text{var}(x - y) = \text{var}(x) + \text{var}(y)$$

Independence can be illustrated with the following examples. Height and weight are not independent, as knowledge of height permits an improved estimate of weight. Obviously the improved estimate is far from perfect, but it is nevertheless better than the estimate possible in the absence of any information. For adults, height and social security number are probably independent, as knowledge of either for any individual is not likely to improve your estimate of the other.

At present we are interested in the variance of the difference between p_c and p_e (sample estimates of P_c and P_e, respectively). In a properly conducted trial, knowledge of the sample result for p_e, e.g., that it was above or below the true value of P_e, would not provide any basis for knowing that in the same trial p_c was above or below the true value of P_c. Thus, the sample data p_e and p_c are independent and

$$\text{var}(p_c - p_e) = \text{var}(p_c) + \text{var}(p_e)$$

We now consider a specific example. What is the sample size needed, with equal numbers of subjects in control and experimental groups, to detect a significant difference between p_e and p_c with a two-sided type I error of .05 (i.e., reject the null hypothesis if the difference between p_e and p_c is large and positive *or* large and negative) and a type II error of .10, if P_c really is .03 and P_e really is .02. Figure 2-1 presents these concepts in nonquantitative form.

Our explanation of sample size calculations rests upon Figures 2-1 through 2-6. If you understand what has been added or changed from each figure to the next, you should have a clear conception of the ideas involved. In Figures 2-1 through 2-6 the total area under each sampling distribution is standardized at unity. Thus, if a labeled area is shown as equal to .025, it can be read as meaning that the *probability* of a sample difference being in that specific area of the distribution is .025.

For our specific example, we need to calculate $\text{var}(p_c - p_e)$ if the null hypothesis is true. Recognizing that in this instance both p_c and p_e represent sample estimates of a parameter of .03 (i.e., P_e is *not* different from P_c, which equals .03), we have

$$\text{var}(d): H_0 = \frac{.03(.97)}{n} + \frac{.03(.97)}{n}$$

where $d = p_c - p_e$ and $\text{var}(d): H_0$ is the variance of the difference under the null hypothesis.

The standard error of the difference $p_c - p_e$ if the null hypothesis is true is the square root of the above:

$$\text{SE}(d): H_0 = \left[\frac{.03(.97)}{n} + \frac{.03(.97)}{n} \right]^{1/2}$$

This formulation is the same as that used to calculate n on the basis of specified confidence limits. However, in order to bring into the calculations the power of our sample size to reject the null hypothesis when a specified alternative is true, we are now considering sample size calculations from the viewpoint of hypothesis testing. Of course, after the data have been collected, presenting results in terms of confidence limits on the unknown difference between the two parameters is always more informative than simply rejecting or not rejecting the null hypothesis.

Recalling that in our test of the null hypothesis we have a two-sided type I error of .05, we can identify the critical value as the point marked "V" in Figure 2-1. This point is 1.96 $\text{SE}(d): H_0$ above the mean value of zero difference, given that the null hypothesis is true. If this is not immediately obvious, consider the following argument. We are investigating two possible states. Either both control and experimental groups have $P = .03$, which is the null hypothesis state, or $P_c = .03$ but $P_e = .02$, which is the alternative hypothesis state. A type I error of size α represents a rejection of the null hypothesis *when it is true*. If the null hypothesis is true, any sample difference falling in the two areas marked $\alpha/2$ will result in falsely rejecting the null hypothesis; for these two symmetric areas to have a total probability of .05, they must each be 1.96 $\text{SE}(d): H_0$ from the mean.

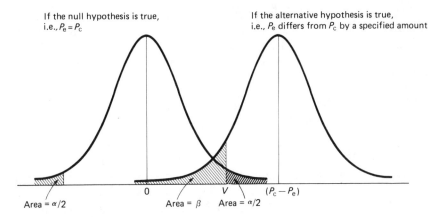

If the null hypothesis is true, i.e., $P_e = P_c$

If the alternative hypothesis is true, i.e., P_e differs from P_c by a specified amount

Area = $\alpha/2$ 0   Area = β V Area = $\alpha/2$ $(P_c - P_e)$

Figure 2-1. Distribution of all possible differences of sample means.

Here again we are making use of characteristics of the normal distribution. For the sample sizes appropriate to epidemiologic studies, the normality assumption is almost always justified.

In Figure 2-2 we repeat Figure 2-1 with some simplifications and an indication that V is 1.96 SE(d): H_0 from the mean (zero) of the distribution of all possible sample differences under the null hypothesis.

Suppose the true state is that of the alternative hypothesis. In that case, sample differences falling in the region to the left of V lead to our failure to reject the null hypothesis when the alternative is true. This is the type II error (of size β), and in this particular example we have set β equal to .10.

Perhaps a better way of thinking about type II error is to state the probability desired for rejecting H_0 when the alternative is true, which is $(1 - \beta)$. If we want this to be .90, then $(1 - \beta) = .90$ and $\beta = .10$.

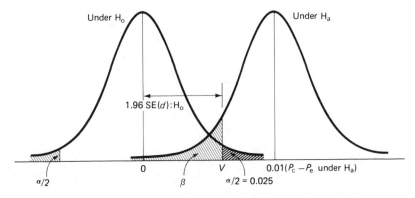

Under H_o Under H_a

1.96 SE(d):H_o

$\alpha/2$ 0 β V $\alpha/2 = 0.025$ 0.01($P_c - P_e$ under H_a)

Figure 2-2. Distribution of all possible differences of sample means with type error (α) set equal to .05.

Again making use of the characteristics of the normal distribution, we know that 10 percent of the tail area on one side of the mean is located beyond 1.28 standard deviations from the mean. In this example the standard deviation of the distribution of all possible sample differences under the alternative hypothesis is

$$SE(d): H_a = \left[\frac{.03(.97)}{n} + \frac{.02(.98)}{n} \right]^{1/2}$$

and we can add to the diagram that V is 1.28 $SE(d): H_a$ from the mean of the distribution of all possible sample differences under the alternative hypothesis. This is shown in Figure 2-3, which can be used to derive a formula for calculating n. Note that 1.96 $SE(d): H_0 + 1.28$ $SE(d): H_a$ equals exactly the distance between the means of the two sampling distributions. Thus we have 1.96 $SE(d): H_0 + 1.28$ $SE(d): H_a = .01$, from which we can calculate n:

$$1.96 \left[\frac{.03(.97)}{n} + \frac{.03(.97)}{n} \right]^{1/2} + 1.28 \left[\frac{.03(.97)}{n} + \frac{.02(.98)}{n} \right]^{1/2} = 0.1$$

$$1.96 \left(\frac{.2412}{\sqrt{n}} \right) + 1.28 \left(\frac{.2207}{\sqrt{n}} \right) = .01$$

$$\sqrt{n} = 75.52$$

$$n = 5703$$

In reviewing the components of this formula, we observe that 1.96 was used for $Z_{\alpha/2}$, the standardized normal deviate appropriate to a one-sided area of $\alpha/2$ (two-sided error $= \alpha$). If the two-sided α is set equal to .01, we use 2.58 instead of 1.96. The value of var $(d): H_0$ represents the variance of the difference between two sample means, both drawn from a binomial universe with $P = P_c$,

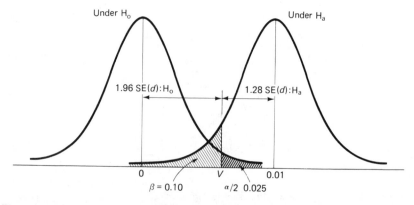

Under H_o Under H_a

1.96 SE(d):H_o 1.28 SE(d):H_a

0   V   0.01

$\beta = 0.10$ $\alpha/2$ 0.025

Figure 2-3. Distribution of all possible differences of sample means with type error (α) set equal to .05 and type II error (β) set equal to .10.

which in this case is .03. The value 1.28 represents the Z_β that is appropriate to the standardized normal deviate beyond which in one direction the proportion β of the distribution lies. If the type II error had been set at .05 instead of .10, Z_β would be 1.64 instead of 1.28. The values used for var(d): H_a represent the variance of the difference of two binomial means, one drawn from a population with $P = .03$ and the other from a population with $P = .02$. I now restate, in general terms, the equation to be solved for sample size n, using Q to represent $1 - P$:

$$Z_{\alpha/2}\left(\frac{2P_cQ_c}{n}\right)^{1/2} + Z_\beta\left(\frac{P_cQ_c}{n} + \frac{P_eQ_e}{n}\right)^{1/2} = P_c - P_e^{\ddagger} \tag{2-6}$$

Most texts, references, and experts [14,15] would argue that the above equation is wrong and that $2P_cQ_c$ should be replaced by $2\overline{PQ}$, where $\overline{P} = (P_c + P_e)/2$. While not agreeing with the majority on this point, I want to present their view. In simplest terms, the disagreement arises because the actual significance test performed *after* data have been collected tests whether the two observed values p_c and p_e could both represent samples from a population whose parameter is $(p_c + p_e)/2$, or $\bar{p}$. I would perform the same test, but my view is that the null hypothesis (to use the arithmetic values from the preceding illustration) states that both parameters are .03 (value of P_c), not that both are .025 $[(P_c + P_e)/2]$. The sampling variance under the null hypothesis follows from the null hypothesis. The sample size calculated from Equation 2-6 is exactly the sample size appropriate to the question "If the true control proportion is P_c and the true experimental proportion Pe, what sample size is needed to be $1 - \beta$ sure of detecting a significant difference at the α level between control and experimental means?" Having computed the sample size appropriate to this question, I shall use the data actually collected to answer a different question: Are p_c and p_e random samples from a binomial universe with $(p_c + p_e)/2$ as mean?

As a practical matter, it is useful to note that this difference of opinion has only a moderate effect on the calculated value of n.

Unrelated to the previous discussion of the correct formula is an approximation to Equation 2-6 which substitutes $\overline{P} = (P_c + P_e)/2$ for both P_c and P_e. Using Δ to represent $P_c - P_e$, this short form becomes

$$Z_{\alpha/2}\left(\frac{2\overline{PQ}}{n}\right)^{1/2} + Z_\beta\left(\frac{2\overline{PQ}}{n}\right)^{1/2} = \Delta$$

$$(Z_{\alpha/2} + Z_\beta)\left(\frac{2\overline{PQ}}{n}\right)^{1/2} = \Delta$$

$$(Z_{\alpha/2} + Z_\beta)^2\left(\frac{2\overline{PQ}}{n}\right) = \Delta^2$$

$$n = \frac{(Z_{\alpha/2} + Z_\beta)^2(2\overline{PQ})}{\Delta^2} \tag{2-7}$$

Unlike Equation 2-6, Equation 2-7 requires an equal number of subjects in both groups. Equation 2-6 is simple to solve for n even if written so that there are n subjects in one group and $2n$ or $3n$ in the other (e.g., for study designs with two or three controls for each case).

Sample size calculations presented herein relate to simple random sampling. For stratified, systematic, or cluster sampling, the same equations are used with full recognition that good stratification or relevant ordering of a list from which a systematic sample is taken will increase precision from that specified and, with few exceptions, cluster sampling will reduce precision from that specified.

All the preceding examples of sample size calculations relate to binomial variables. Exactly the same principles apply to continuous variables (e.g., blood pressure or weight) with $\text{var}(X)$ substituted for $P(1 - P)$ and μ for P. Equation 2-4 rewritten for a continuous variable becomes

$$1.96 \ SE(\bar{x}) = 1.96 \left[\frac{\text{var}(X)}{n} \right]^{1/2} = \Delta \tag{2-8}$$

where Δ equals the difference between estimate and parameter that we are willing to tolerate. Equation 2-5 rewritten for a continuous variable becomes

$$1.96 \ SE(\bar{x}) = 1.96 \left[\frac{\text{var}(X)}{n} \right]^{1/2} = \frac{\mu}{K} \tag{2-9}$$

Equation 2-6 rewritten for a comparison of continuous variables, with X representing the result of standard treatment and Y the result of experimental treatment, becomes

$$Z_{\alpha/2} \left[\frac{2\text{var}(X)}{n} \right]^{1/2} + Z_{\beta} \left[\frac{\text{var}(X)}{n} + \frac{\text{var}(Y)}{n} \right]^{1/2} = \mu_x - \mu_y \, \S \tag{2-10}$$

For continuous variables it is entirely possible that $\text{var}(X) = \text{var}(Y)$ even though $\mu_x \neq \mu_y$. For binomial variables, if means differ, so must the variances, as they are directly related.

Estimates of the variances required for calculating sample size appropriate for the study of continuous variables must depend on prior data and on the investigator's informed judgment.

It may be helpful for students to consider the effect of different sizes of n on the distribution of all possible sample differences, as shown in Figures 2-1 to 2-3. First let us imagine how the distributions might look if n were very large, thus reducing the size of both $SE(d)$: H_0 and $SE(d)$: H_a, but without changing the location of V. This is shown in Figure 2-4, wherein both $\alpha/2$ and β are smaller than in Figures 2-1 to 2-3.

Suppose (as is traditional) that, despite the larger sample size, α is kept

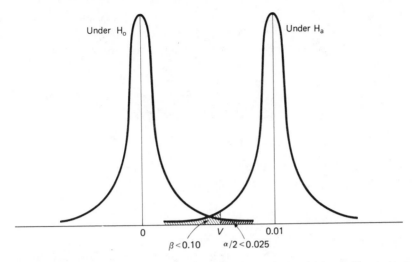

Figure 2-4. Distribution of all possible differences of sample means if sample size is very large.

constant at .05 and $\alpha/2$ at .025. Then the distributions for very large n would look like Figure 2-5, in which V' is the critical value above which we make a type I error if the null hypothesis is true and below which we make a type II error if the alternative hypothesis is true. The cross-hatched area immediately to the right of V' represents $\alpha/2 = .025$ of the total area under the distribution, given H_0. Note how much *farther V' is from the mean of the distribution under the alternative hypothesis* relative to our original critical value, V. As a

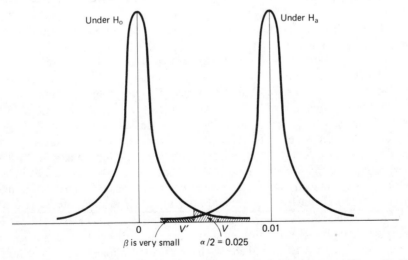

Figure 2-5. Distribution of all possible differences of sample means if sample size is very large but type I error (α) is kept equal to .05.

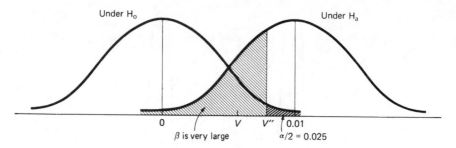

Figure 2-6. Distribution of all possible differences of sample means if sample size is *not* large and type I error (α) is kept equal to .05.

consequence, the probability of a type II error has been drastically reduced. If in fact the alternative hypothesis is true, we have very little chance of failing to reject the null hypothesis ($\beta < .01$, estimated from Figure 2-5).

Next look at Figure 2-6, in which we consider the effect on the two distributions of a small n (but still large enough to justify our use of the normal curve for the distribution of all possible sample differences). Again the two-sided α is fixed at .05.

Now V'' is the critical value above which we make a type I error if the null hypothesis is true. This error is again fixed at .05 (two-sided), but observe how large β has become. Since for values of $p_c - p_e$ below (to the left of) V'' we do not reject the null hypothesis, Figure 2-6 shows that we shall be doing this about 25 percent of the time that samples are actually taken from the universe specified by the alternative hypothesis. To review, Figures 2-4, 2-5, and 2-6 show that for a fixed type I error, the probability of failing to reject the null hypothesis when the alternative is true (β) will be small for large samples and large for small samples.

A final note about sample size. Sample size calculations are needed to ensure that the study design is adequate for at least some question of interest. As a practical matter, there are always subsidiary questions of importance. Furthermore, some individuals assigned to a treatment will refuse, and others may not adhere to the schedule of treatment or be lost to follow-up. All these factors reduce the effect that can be observed. Experienced investigators know that sample size, however calculated, is invariably inadequate for some purposes. Some methods of analysis, such as matching or multiple adjustment, tend to reduce the variance of sample statistics and thus to reduce the sample size needed to a value lower than that obtained by using Equations 2-4 to 2-10. Unfortunately, this favorable influence is more than balanced by the increased sample size necessary for subgroup comparisons. I advise the use of Equations 2-4 to 2-10, modified when necessary by inclusion of the finite sampling factor, together with an appreciation that the resultant sample size usually reflects minimum needs.

NOTES

* To check that no possibilities have been omitted, we can calculate the number of combinations of eight elements taken two at a time. The first element selected could be any one of the eight, and for each of these there are seven possible ways of picking the second selection. Thus, there are 56 different possibilities for selecting two from eight, but these include permutations, such $0_a 0_b$ and $0_b 0_a$. Since in either case exactly the same two elements make up the sample, the order in which they were chosen is unimportant to us and they are alike for our purpose. To reduce the 56 permutations to combinations that involve different elements, we need only divide by the possible number of permutations of two things, which is 2. Thus $56 \div 2 = 28$ different samples of two, in agreement with the direct count.

† There are only 16 possible different stratified samples of size 2, as compared to 28 for simple sampling. The total of 16 can be checked as follows. If we pick from stratum 1 four choices are possible and for *each* of these four choices are possible from stratum 2, the total is 16. Picking first from stratum 2 only introduces permutations of the 16 samples already cited. Since we are interested in different samples and not in the order of choosing sample elements, these permutations can be ignored.

‡ Depending on the direction of the change expected from the experimental treatment, this should be written $P_c - P_e$ or $P_e - P_c$, whichever shows a positive difference.

§ This should be written $\mu_x - \mu_y$ or $\mu_y - \mu_x$, whichever reflects a positive difference.

3

Relative Risk and Odds Ratio

Since Cornfield showed that under suitable conditions retrospective studies* can provide estimates of relative risk [16], this statistic (as well as the odds ratio, which is closely related to it) has been used extensively in epidemiologic investigations as a measure of strength of association between a disease and a risk factor. Although, for reasons to be discussed later, I prefer the odds ratio, for historical reasons the discussion begins with relative risk.

RELATIVE RISK

Consider a population followed prospectively as described in Table 3-1. The risk of disease developing among those with the risk factor is $A/(A + B)$. Similarly, the risk of disease developing among those without the risk factor is $C/(C + D)$. The risk for those with the risk factor relative to those without the risk factor is the ratio of the two risks, $\dfrac{A/(A + B)}{C/(C + D)}$. Although relative risk could be calculated and reported for a prospective study, often it is not. In prospective studies, emphasis is rightly placed on the direct assessment of risk for various

Table 3-1. Classification of a Population by Risk Factor Status and Disease Development in an Incidence Study

Risk factor classification	Disease incidence		Total at risk
	+	−	
+ (present)	A	B	A + B
− (absent)	C	D	C + D
Total	A + C	B + D	T

groups and relative risk is not likely to be a prominent component of the analysis. For retrospective studies, however, direct assessment of risk for specific groups is often impossible and the estimation of relative risk assumes major importance. Before proceeding to the mechanics of relative risk estimation in retrospective studies, we shall briefly review the logical foundations for obtaining relative risk in such studies.

Logical Basis for Retrospective Studies

The most basic requirement for obtaining relative risk estimates from retrospective studies is that the cases in the study be representative of all the cases under consideration and that the controls in the study be representative of all the noncases under consideration. The word *representative* refers to representativeness *with respect to the risk factors being evaluated*. The term *under consideration* refers to the population being studied.

Suppose that both cases and controls are taken from a private hospital principally used by patients in high socioeconomic categories. If the intent is to study the disease-risk factor association in this upper-class subpopulation, restricting cases and controls to such a hospital can be defended. If the intent is to study the risk-disease association in the total population, the restriction to private hospital data may be challenged. Evidence may exist establishing that risk does not vary by social class, but more likely the applicability to the total population of findings based on a particular subpopulation would be unknown. Although it is unlikely that the study cases and controls will have the identical proportion with the risk factor as all cases and all noncases, respectively, strong bias must be absent. Sampling error, although always present, is not a fundamental difficulty because it is controllable with adequate sample size. However, if cases are selected so that the method of selection produces important differences from all cases—and similarly for controls relative to all noncases—then it is quite possible that the proportion with the risk factor among *cases in the study* will differ by much more than sampling error from the proportion with the risk factor among *all relevant cases*. Details regarding selection of cases and controls are discussed in many texts on epidemiology [8,17–19], but the essential requirement is the one stated above.

While prospective studies can estimate the relative risk with respect to becoming sick (incident cases), retrospective studies can estimate only the relative risk with respect to being sick (prevalent cases). The practical importance of this distinction ranges from trivial to enormous. The retrospective study that compares existing cases with noncases (controls) on one or more potential risk factors cannot, in principle, relate to all cases occurring (incident) during the past *n* years because some of these incident cases may no longer be alive. The prospective study can, in principle, relate to all incident cases, whether early deaths or not, because risk factor status is measured at the onset of observation. For a disease such as myocardial infarction, in which a large fraction die promptly upon the very first clinical manifestation of the disease, relative risks derived from retrospective studies *may* be quite different from those obtained in prospective studies. *If* early myocardial infarction deaths are unrepresentative of the myocardial infarction prevalent cases with respect to the risk factor being investigated, the difference can be great. Furthermore, a retrospective study tends to identify factors related to improved survival as risk factors for being sick. On the other hand, relative risk for a disease such as senile cataract, which is not associated with increased mortality risk, is, in principle, equally estimable in prospective and retrospective studies.

A second major qualification for retrospective studies to be able to provide estimates of relative risk equivalent to those from a prospective study relates to when risk factor information is collected. In prospective studies, these data are collected prior to the development of disease and thus cannot be influenced or biased by disease status. (The possibility that ascertainment of disease in a prospective study may be biased by knowledge of risk factor status is a separate problem to be guarded against in study procedures.) In retrospective studies, risk factor data are collected after disease status is known and are subject to potential bias for that reason. Similar to differences arising from the use of incident or prevalent cases, the practical consequences of this potential problem vary greatly depending on the specific disease and risk factor under consideration. To illustrate, Table 3-2 lists several specific risk factors, in relation to myocardial infarction, showing a range of potential measurement bias from nonexistent to major.

Investigators conducting retrospective studies must be aware of these (and other) potential biases. The final logical requirement for a successful retrospective study is that data collection methods for risk factors be similar for

Table 3-2. Illustration of Bias Potential in Retrospective Study Measurement of Risk Factors for Myocardial Infarction

Risk factor	Potential measurement bias due to measuring *after* disease status is known
Age began smoking	It is possible that those with the disease may try harder than controls to recall correctly an event of many years past.
Current smoking	Obvious major bias since myocardial infarction patients are almost always forbidden to smoke by attending physician. Current smoking probably does not reflect the risk factor intended for study. This is typically avoided by changing the risk factor from "current smoking" to smoking habits of "a month ago," "a year ago," "prior to your illness," etc.
Years of education completed	It is possible that those with the disease may be more (or less) given to exaggeration about a variable of social importance. However, for this variable the possibility exists of locating official records, thereby completely eliminating measurement bias.
Blood type	Bias is nonexistent for any objectively measurable genetic trait.

Table 3-3. Association of Risk Factors and Disease in a
Retrospective Study Sample

Risk factor classification	Cases	Controls	Total
+ (present)	a	b	m_1
− (absent)	c	d	m_2
Total	$a + c = n_1$	$b + d = n_2$	$m_1 + m_2 = t$

cases and controls. If risk factor data for cases come from relatives of cases, so should data for controls. If risk factor data for cases come from records, so should data for controls. If risk factor data are obtained by interviewers, the same interviewers should contact both cases and controls, without knowledge as to which is which, insofar as this is possible.

Estimation of Association from Sample Data

Assuming that we have conducted a retrospective study and chosen study cases and controls so as to represent all cases and all noncases in the population being investigated, have avoided measurement bias due to differences in data collection methods between cases and controls, have minimized bias due to risk factor measurement after disease has developed, and have been able to rule out important differences in risk factor frequency between incident cases and prevalent cases, we can summarize study results as in Table 3-3.

Frequently, $b + d$ is chosen to equal $a + c$, that is, the total number of controls equals the total number of cases. Since the number of cases and the number of controls are usually determined *without knowledge* of how many cases and how many noncases actually exist in the population of interest, it is impossible to use any ratio of cases to controls to reflect the risk for a specific group. The ratio $a/(a + b)$, for example, does *not* estimate the risk of disease for those with the risk factor. This ratio is in fact useless by itself.

The key to understanding how the data in Table 3-3 can be used to estimate relative risk is in recognizing that $a + c$ is a sample of total cases and $b + d$ is a separate sample of noncases. Thus, although the relationship of a to b or a to $a + b$ promises no meaningful data (since it reflects in part decisions such as having one or two controls per case), the relationship of a to c provides an estimate of how all cases are divided into those with and without the risk factor. Similarly, whereas the ratios c/d and $c/(c + d)$ are usually uninterpretable, the ratio b/d estimates the distribution of the risk factor among all noncases.

Table 3-4 cross-classifies the total population from which the cases and controls in Table 3-3 were selected, and a/c and b/d in Table 3-3 can be interpreted as estimates of A/C and B/D in Table 3-4. Thus, while we cannot estimate the risk of disease for those with and without the risk factor, we can estimate how the risk factor is distributed among those with and without disease.

Table 3-4. Association of Risk Factor and Disease in a Population Cross Section

Risk factor classification	Cases	Noncases	Total
+ (present)	A	B	M_1
− (absent)	C	D	M_2
Total	$A + C = N_1$	$B + D = N_2$	$M_1 + M_2 = T$

I now use Table 3-4 to explain how the retrospective study data a/c and b/d can be used to estimate relative risk. Analagous to what has been stated for incidence, the relative risk of having disease for those with compared with those without the risk factor is $\dfrac{A/(A+B)}{C/(C+D)}$. This ratio referred to Table 3-1 definitions is the relative risk of *becoming* sick; with reference to Table 3-4 definitions, it is the relative risk of *being* sick. For diseases that are uncommon, and happily for humanity many diseases fit this requirement, $A + B$ can usually be satisfactorily approximated by B. Similarly, $C + D$ can usually be approximated by D. Making these substitutions, we have:

$$\frac{A/(A+B)}{C/(C+D)} \simeq \frac{A/B}{C/D} = \frac{AD}{BC} \tag{3-1}$$

To repeat, if the disease is rare *in the population* (how common or rare it is in the sample studied depends on how many controls were selected per case), the relative risk is closely approximated by AD/BC, commonly called the *odds ratio*. The odds ratio can also be defined directly, rather than as something approximately equal to the relative risk under certain conditions, and we now do so.

ODDS RATIO

The distinction between risk and odds can be illustrated using the notation of Table 3-4, where $A/(A + B)$ is the *risk* of disease among those with the risk factor and A/B is the *odds* of disease to nondisease among those with the risk factor. The application of odds that might be familiar to most readers relates to gambling. Odds of 2 to 1 are equivalent to a probability of 2 out of 3. Odds of 5 to 2 are equivalent to a probability of 5 out of 7. Odds thus have the same numerators as probabilities, but the denominators count only those events not counted in the numerator. The denominator of a probability is always a count of all relevant events, including those counted in the numerator. If in Table 3-4 A has the value 1 and B the value 99, the risk of disease for those with the risk factor would be 1/100 and the odds of disease to nondisease for those with the risk factor would be 1/99.

Again referring to Table 3-4, the odds ratio relating the *odds of being a case to not being a case* for those with the risk factor (A/B) to these same odds for those without the risk factor (C/D) is $(A/B)/(C/D)$, which has just been shown to be a good approximation to the relative risk for uncommon diseases. Interestingly, the other odds ratio obtainable from Table 3-4, i.e., relating the *odds of having or not having the risk factor* for those who are cases (A/C) to these same odds for those who are not cases (B/D) also equals $(A/B)/(C/D)$. This is easy to see:

$$\frac{A/C}{B/D} = \frac{A}{C}\left(\frac{D}{B}\right) = \frac{A}{B}\left(\frac{D}{C}\right) = \frac{A/B}{C/D} \qquad (3\text{-}2)$$

The odds ratio is usually reported in its simplest form, which is AD/BC. However, the algebraic equivalents of AD/BC, $(A/C)/(B/D)$, or $(A/B)/(C/D)$ express the odds in the numerator and denominator of the ratio more clearly than does AD/BC.

If instead of population data in Table 3-4, we make use of sample data in Table 3-3 to calculate odds ratios, as we previously explained, we are not able to use a/b or c/d as estimates of the odds for disease to nondisease in the population. However, we can and do use a/c and b/d as estimates of the population odds for having, relative to not having, the risk factor. As shown in Equation 3-2, however, the ratios $(A/C)/(B/D)$ and $(A/B)/(C/D)$ are identically equal to AD/BC, the population odds ratio.

Arrangement of 2 × 2 Tables

At this point, a brief digression concerning the ordering of rows and columns in 2 × 2 tables may be helpful. Note that both Tables 3-3 and 3-4 are arranged so that data for those *with* the risk factor is in the first row and data for cases is in the first column. Often, locating data for those with the risk factor in the first row is contrary to natural numeric ordering. For example, the first row might contain data for those with higher blood pressure and the second row data for those with lower blood pressure. This is done deliberately. Consider the symbolic sample data arrangement in Table 3-3. Under the proper conditions of sampling and measurement, ad/bc estimates the ratio in the population of the odds of being a case for those with the factor present, to the odds of being a case for those with the factor absent. This particular odds ratio is no more correct than the other odds ratio that can be estimated from these data; it is just customary and convenient for the odds ratio to be in this form. In Table 3-4, AD/BC is the odds of being a case for those with the factor present (A/B) divided by the odds of being a case for those with the factor absent (C/D). In sample data arranged the same way, ad/bc provides an estimate of AD/BC.

If both the population and the sample data in Tables 3-3 and 3-4 had been arranged so that the first row of the table was "risk factor absent" and the second row was "risk factor present" but with the A-B-C-D and a-b-c-d labeling for the four cells unchanged, then AD/BC would represent the odds of being a case for those *with factor absent* (A/B) divided by the odds of being a case for those *with factor present* (C/D). Thus with this changed ordering of the data, calculating ad/bc from the sample estimates a population odds ratio different from the one estimated from an identical sample 2×2 table but with row data reversed. If presence of the factor raises the risk of disease, then AD/BC from Table 3-4 will have a value greater than unity and AD/BC from a table similar to Table 3-4 but with row data reversed will have a value less than unity. There are only two odds ratios definable from a 2×2 table, and each is the reciprocal of the other. Returning to Table 3-4 notation, the possibility for calculating odds in terms of *disease* are A/B and C/D or B/A and D/C. The odds ratios possible are odds for those with factor present divided by odds for those with factor absent and odds for those with factor absent divided by odds for those with factor present. The possibilities for calculating odds in terms of *risk factors* are A/C and B/D or C/A and D/B. In this instance, the odds ratio could relate odds for those with disease to odds for those without disease or odds for those without disease to odds for those with disease. Using all possible combinations, we get

$$\frac{A/B}{C/D} = \frac{AD}{BC} \qquad \frac{B/A}{D/C} = \frac{BC}{AD} \qquad \frac{A/C}{B/D} = \frac{AD}{BC} \qquad \frac{C/A}{D/B} = \frac{BC}{AD}$$

$$\frac{C/D}{A/B} = \frac{BC}{AD} \qquad \frac{D/C}{B/A} = \frac{AD}{BC} \qquad \frac{B/D}{A/C} = \frac{BC}{AD} \qquad \frac{D/B}{C/A} = \frac{AD}{BC}$$

It is always essential to know what you are doing with respect to summarization of data, but it is still convenient to be able to use the routine calculation of a cross-product ratio, ad/bc, in obtaining an estimate of the odds ratio of interest. Recognizing that reversing the two rows (or the two columns) of the table leads to estimating the reciprocal odds ratio often helps identify any instances when the table is arranged in a manner other than intended. (Reversing both rows *and* columns of the table leads to inverting an inverted ratio, which leaves it unchanged.)

A final comment on row and column ordering. The cross-product ratio ad/bc is affected by which of the two rows is on top and which of the two columns is on the left. Having fixed these, whether the disease-nondisease data are in rows and the risk factor data in columns or vice versa does not affect the cross-product ratio.

Odds Ratio Review

To recapitulate, a properly designed and conducted case control study:

1. Provides no data on disease odds separately for risk factor groups.
2. Does provide estimates of risk factor odds separately for cases and noncases. For Table 3-3, this is a/c and b/d.

3. Provides an estimate, ad/bc, of the population odds ratio, AD/BC, which for rare diseases (perhaps prevalence less than .05) is a good approximation of the population relative risk $\dfrac{A/(A + B)}{C/(C + D)}$.

One aspect of using retrospective study data to estimate relative risk that seems inadequately understood is that the sample data, ad/bc, are *always* usable as an estimator of the population odds ratio, AD/BC, whether or not the disease is rare in the population. When the disease is rare, AD/BC is sufficiently close to $\dfrac{A/(A + B)}{C/(C + D)}$ to make ad/bc an estimate of relative risk as well as the odds ratio. Since odds are not as much a part of ordinary usage as chance or probability or risk, many people find the concept of an odds ratio less meaningful than a relative risk. I think this is a matter of custom rather than of basic superiority of one method over the other and that odds and odds ratios will be increasingly used by epidemiologists in the future.

An Odds Ratio Advantage

One aspect of the odds ratio that is superior to the relative risk is the former's insensitivity to whether a study stresses death or survival. This point is illustrated by Table 3-5. Using Table 3-5 data to compare community A with community B, the relative risk of dying is $(2/100) \div (1/100) = 2$. The same comparison of odds leads to the odds ratio $(2/98) \div (1/99) \cong 2$. Thus, both measures indicate double or about double the risk of dying in community A relative to community B.

We now use Table 3-5 data to compare the two communities, but this time with respect to *surviving* instead of dying. The relative "risk" for surviving is $(98/100) \div (99/100) \cong 1$. The odds ratio for surviving is $(98/2) \div (99/1) \cong 1/2$. The use of relative risk leads to different results depending on whether the study is summarized with respect to death or to survival. Using the odds ratio, however, it does not really matter. Community A has about twice the odds of community B with respect to dying and about half the odds of community B with respect to surviving. This indifference as to whether stress is placed on counting the events or the nonevents is obviously a desirable property of a summary statistic. The odds ratio has this property, the relative risk does not.

Table 3-5. Comparison of Mortality Experience in Two Communities

Community	Number dying	Number surviving	Total
A	2	98	100
B	1	99	100
Total	3	197	200

RELATIVE RISK FROM RETROSPECTIVE STUDIES

It is sometimes claimed that retrospective studies can estimate relative risk only for rare diseases because it is only for rare diseases that the population relative risk is approximated by the population odds ratio. While this is frequently true as a practical consequence of how retrospective studies are conducted, exceptions are possible. I shall use the notation of Tables 3-3 and 3-4 to make this point.

If, as is rarely done, controls are selected not to represent noncases but to represent the *total population* (for example, selecting an area sample for controls), the relative risk can be estimated without regard to disease rarity. The study data in this instance, a/c and b/d, would estimate A/C and $(A + B)/(C + D)$, respectively. The ratio $(a/c) \div (b/d)$ would then estimate $\dfrac{A/(A + B)}{C/(C + D)}$ whether or not the disease is rare. Since controls are rarely samples of the total population, the usual rule that retrospective studies can estimate relative risk only for rare diseases is correct. If, however, controls do represent the total population rather than just noncases, this need not be. Again, we emphasize that whether or not the disease is rare, $(a/c) \div (b/d)$, where $b + d$ is a sample of noncases, is an appropriate estimator of AD/BC, the odds ratio in the population.

CONFIDENCE LIMITS FOR ODDS RATIOS

We shall use OR as a symbol for AD/BC in the population and $\widehat{OR}$ as a symbol for an estimate of OR based on sample data. For data as in Table 3-3, the odds ratio is estimated as $\widehat{OR} = ad/bc$. To obtain 95 percent confidence limits on OR using Woolf's method [20], we calculate $\ln \widehat{OR}$ and its estimated standard error:

$$\text{SE}(\ln \widehat{OR}) = \left(\frac{1}{a} + \frac{1}{b} + \frac{1}{c} + \frac{1}{d}\right)^{1/2} \tag{3-3}$$

Then 95 percent confidence limits on $\ln OR$ are

$$\ln \widehat{OR} \pm 1.96 \left(\frac{1}{a} + \frac{1}{b} + \frac{1}{c} + \frac{1}{d}\right)^{1/2}$$

For 99 percent confidence limits, substitute 2.58 for 1.96. When confidence limits on $\ln OR$ have been obtained, confidence limits on OR are derived by taking antilogs. If $\ln OR_U$ and $\ln OR_L$ are the upper and lower confidence limits for $\ln OR$, then $e^{\ln OR_U}$ and $e^{\ln OR_L}$ are the upper and lower confidence limits for OR.

Some authors advocate the addition of 1/2 to each of the cell frequencies $a, b, c,$ and d before calculation of $\widehat{OR}$ or of SE $\ln \widehat{OR}$ [21, 22]. Others do not

Table 3-6. Relationship of Cataract and Diabetes in a Case-Control Study, Age 50 to 69

Diabetes	Cataract cases	Fracture patients (controls)
+ (present)	55	84
− (absent)	552	1927

Source: R. A. Hiller and H. A. Kahn, *Br. J. Ophthalmol.* **60**:283 (1976).

use the 1/2 adjustment or have reservations concerning it [23, 24]. I make no recommendation about this except to emphasize two points. First, if any cell frequency is zero, it may be impossible to carry out the calculations outlined in this and later chapters unless the 1/2 is added. Second, epidemiologic studies summarized into 2×2 tables with cell totals of zero or with cell totals so small that adding 1/2 will substantially affect the summary calculations are rarely of adequate precision to contribute anything of importance to our knowledge.

To illustrate the use of Woolf's method in calculating 95 percent confidence limits on OR, we apply the method to the data in Table 3-6, taken from a case-control study on the relationship of cataract to diabetes [25].

$$\hat{OR} = \frac{55(1927)}{84(552)} = 2.29$$

$$\ln \hat{OR} = .8286$$

$$SE(\ln \hat{OR}) = \left(\frac{1}{55} + \frac{1}{1927} + \frac{1}{84} + \frac{1}{552} \right)^{1/2} = .1800$$

$$\ln \hat{OR} \pm 1.96\,SE(\ln \hat{OR}) = .8286 \pm .3528$$

95 percent CL on $\ln OR$ = .4758 and 1.1814

95 percent CL on $OR = e^{.4758}$ and $e^{1.1814}$ = 1.6 and 3.3

These same data were used to calculate confidence limits on the odds ratio using Cornfield's method as reported by Gart [26]. That method, which requires an iterative procedure, is not as convenient as Woolf's method but is generally acknowledged to be more accurate. In this instance, however, the more accurate method makes no difference. The 95 percent confidence limits derived from the above data using Cornfield's method are also 1.6 and 3.3. In order to compare the two methods when the 2×2 table has cells of much smaller size, we make use of additional data reported by Hiller and Kahn for subgroups [25]. The resultant confidence limits are shown in Table 3-7. Although the size of the smallest cell is smaller in Table 3-7 than in Table 3-6, differences between the two methods are not large, and Woolf's method can be properly said to provide results very similar to those from the more precise method. As shown in Chapter 5, the methods outlined in this book for

Table 3-7. Comparison of 95% Confidence Limits on Odds Ratio Relating Cataract and Diabetes for Various Race and Control Groups, Age 50 to 69

Race	Control diagnoses*	$\hat{OR}$	95% CL on OR Cornfield [26]	Woolf [20]	In 2×2 table, size of smallest Cell	Row or column total
All races	Hemorrhoids	2.1	1.1–4:2	1.1–4.0	12	67
All races	Varicose veins	3.6	1.8–7.4	1.9–6.9	11	66
White	Fractures	2.0	0.9–4.5	1.0–4.2	9	61
Non-white	Fractures	2.2	1.1–4.7	1.1–4.4	13	45

* Presumably reflecting the nondiabetic population.
Source: R. A. Hiller and H. A. Kahn, *Br. J. Ophthalmol.* **60**: 283 (1976).

calculating confidence limits on odds ratios differ to an important extent only when the data do not support a clear inference. However, for those desiring the greater precision of Cornfield's method, see Gart [26].

CONFIDENCE LIMITS FOR RELATIVE RISK

Odds ratios are now more commonly encountered in published reports than direct estimates of relative risk. However, if the individual risks are low enough for the observed events to be treated as Poisson variables, then the number of observed events contains all the relevant information and approximate confidence limits can be computed without great difficulty [27]. The approach outlined below should be reasonably satisfactory for risks less than .10. Let

o_1 represent observed events in sample group 1

o_2 represent observed events in sample group 2

n_1 represent the population size or person-years of observation in sample group 1

n_2 represent the population size or person-years of observation in sample group 2

Then

$$\hat{RR} = \frac{o_1/n_1}{o_2/n_2} = \left(\frac{o_1}{o_2}\right)\left(\frac{n_2}{n_1}\right) \tag{3-4}$$

The confidence limits we shall derive relate only to samples of size n_1 and n_2 with *the sum of the actually observed events* equal to $o_1 + o_2$. The reasons for this can be clarified by imagining the distribution of all possible sample values of o_1 and o_2 arising from all possible samples of size n_1 and n_2. Of all the possible sample outcomes, our attention is restricted to those in which the sum of observed events equals the $o_1 + o_2$ sum in our actual sample. This amounts to taking a slice of the set of all possible samples, but it is a slice that permits inclusion of very large or very small observed values of relative risk. Restricting interest to this set of results enormously simplifies the calculation of the sampling error. We first place confidence limits on the parameter P, which represents the true proportion of the events that are in group 1. Then we use the confidence limits on P to derive confidence limits on the parameter RR, which is our objective.

Sample data can be summarized in the binomial variable

$$p = \frac{o_1}{o_1 + o_2} \tag{3-5}$$

As a binomial variable based on a fixed number of trials (remember that $o_1 + o_2$ is constant over all samples under consideration) and using Equation 1-16, the sampling variance of p can be written

$$\text{var}(p) = \frac{P(1 - P)}{o_1 + o_2}$$

If our data set is large enough to justify using the normal approximation (see [27] if it is not), our sample result of p will be within $1.96[P(1 - P)/n]^{1/2}$ of P 95 percent of the time. In fact, the lowest value of P for which *the observed data would not be unusual* (at the .025 level) is

$$P_L = p - 1.96[P_L(1 - P_L)/(o_1 + o_2)]^{1/2} \tag{3-6}$$

We denote this lower 95 percent confidence limit for P by the symbol P_L.

Another way of stating the relationship shown in Equation 3-6 is that p will not be greater than $P + 1.96\,[SE(p)]$ unless p happens to be one of those unusually large sample values that occur in only 2.5 percent of all possible samples under consideration. Similar reasoning with respect to unusually small sample values of p, which occur in only 2.5 percent of all possible samples under consideration, leads to:

$$P_U = p + 1.96\left[\frac{P_U(1 - P_U)}{o_1 + o_2}\right]^{1/2} \tag{3-7}$$

where P_U is the upper 95 percent confidence limit for P. Since we have found parameter values compatible with p being unusually large or unusually small at the .025 level, solving Equations 3-6 and 3-7 results in 95 percent confidence limits for P. Note that in both Equations the standard error of p is given in terms of P (not p) so that in solving for the upper confidence limit the standard error is based on P_U and in solving for the lower confidence limit the standard error is based on P_L.

We now divide numerator and denominator of Equation 3-4 by $(o_1 + o_2)$ and define the estimated relative risk in terms of the observed binomial proportion p from Equation 3-5:

$$\hat{RR} = \frac{o_1}{o_2}\left(\frac{n_2}{n_1}\right) = \frac{o_1/(o_1 + o_2)}{o_2/(o_1 + o_2)}\left(\frac{n_2}{n_1}\right) = \frac{p}{1-p}\left(\frac{n_2}{n_1}\right) \tag{3-8}$$

If we substitute $\dfrac{P}{1-P}$ for $\dfrac{p}{1-p}$, we have the true relative risk:

$$RR = \frac{P}{1-P}\left(\frac{n_2}{n_1}\right) \tag{3-9}$$

The confidence limits on P relate to confidence limits on RR in the following way. If P is at its .025 lower limit P_L, then $1 - P_L$ is at its .025 upper limit and $P_L/(1 - P_L)$ *will be at its* .025 *lower limit*. Also, if P is at its .025 upper limit P_U, then $(1 - P_U)$ will be at its .025 lower limit and $P_U/(1 - P_U)$ *will be at its* .025 *upper limit*. Thus the limits we have identified for P permit us to calculate confidence limits for RR as well:

$$RR_L = \frac{P_L}{1 - P_L}\left(\frac{n_2}{n_1}\right) \tag{3-10}$$

$$RR_U = \frac{P_U}{1 - P_U}\left(\frac{n_2}{n_1}\right) \tag{3-11}$$

All that remains is to solve Equations 3-6 and 3-7. Since these are quadratic equations, they need to be put into the standard form, $ax^2 + bx + c = 0$ and then solved for x using the formula

$$x = \frac{-b \pm \sqrt{b^2 - 4ac}}{2a}$$

We shall use the data on the 16-year incidence of myocardial infarction in Framingham by serum cholesterol level [28], shown in Table 3-8, to illustrate these computations, first for P_L and then for P_U. Substituting Table 3-8 data into Equaton 3-6, we have

$$P_L = \frac{10}{10 + 21} - 1.96\sqrt{\frac{P_L(1 - P_L)}{10 + 21}}$$

$$P_L - .323 = -1.96\sqrt{\frac{P_L(1 - P_L)}{31}} \tag{3-12}$$

Squaring both sides of the equation, we get

$$P_L^2 - .646\,P_L + .104 = 3.842 \left[\frac{P_L(1 - P_L)}{31} \right]$$

which in standard form is

$$34.842\,P_L^2 - 23.868\,P_L + 3.224 = 0$$

The coefficients of this standard quadratic equation are

$$a = 34.842$$
$$b = -23.868$$
$$c = 3.224$$

so that

$$P_L = \frac{23.868 \pm \sqrt{569.681 - 4(34.842)(3.224)}}{69.684}$$

$$P_L = \frac{34.839}{69.684} \text{ or } \frac{12.897}{69.684} = .500 \text{ or } .185$$

as the two solutions to our quadratic equation. Clearly our choice for the lower limit is .185. However, the .500 is also of interest to us, as we shall soon see.

To solve for the upper limit, we substitute Table 3-8 data into equation 3-7:

$$P_U = \frac{10}{10 + 21} + 1.96 \sqrt{\frac{P_U(1 - P_U)}{10 + 21}}$$

$$P_U - .323 = 1.96 \sqrt{\frac{P_U(1 - P_U)}{31}} \tag{3-13}$$

The only difference between Equation 3-12, which was solved for P_L, and Equation 3-13, which is to be solved for P_U, is $+ 1.96$ or $- 1.96$. Therefore by squaring both sides of Equation 3-13, we obtain the identical quadratic equation obtained for P_L. Since the solutions to that were .185 and .500, we do not need to solve the equation again. This time we take .500, the higher value, as the value for P_U.

Now we apply our values of P_L and P_U to finding limits within which the true relative risk is likely to be found. First, we substitute Table 3-8 data into Equation 3-4 and get

$$\hat{RR} = \frac{10/135}{21/470} = 1.66$$

Then, substituting our P_L and P_U values in Equations 3-10 and 3-11, we get

$$RR_L = \frac{P_L}{1 - P_L}\left(\frac{n_2}{n_1}\right) = \frac{.185}{1 - .185}\left(\frac{470}{135}\right) = .79$$

$$RR_U = \frac{P_U}{1 - P_U}\left(\frac{n_2}{n_1}\right) = \frac{.500}{1 - .500}\left(\frac{470}{135}\right) = 3.48$$

The wide confidence limits (0.79 and 3.48) of the relative risk (1.66) are a necessary consequence of the small total number (31) of observed cases of myocardial infarction.

Recalling that the relative risk and the odds ratios are quite similar for rare diseases and noting that Table 3-8 data reflect 16-year incident data of $10/135 = .074$ for those with high cholesterol levels and $21/470 = .045$ for those with low cholesterol levels, we use Table 3-8 data to calculate the estimated odds ratio and 95 percent confidence limits (by Woolf's method) on the true odds ratio, as an interesting comparison:

$$\hat{OR} = \frac{10(449)}{125(21)} = 1.71$$

$$\ln \hat{OR} = .5368$$

$$SE(\ln \hat{OR}) = \left(\frac{1}{10} + \frac{1}{125} + \frac{1}{21} + \frac{1}{449}\right)^{1/2} = .3973$$

$$1.96\, SE(\ln \hat{OR}) = .7787$$

$$\ln \hat{OR} \pm 1.96\, SE(\ln \hat{OR}) = -.2419 \text{ and } 1.3155 \ (95\% \text{ CL on } \ln OR)$$

$$e^{-.2419} \text{ and } e^{1.3155} = .79 \text{ and } 3.73 \ (95\% \text{ CL on } OR)$$

These compare quite well with the corresponding values for the relative risk.

It should be noted that agreement between relative risk and odds ratio based on longitudinal data can always be increased by shortening the observation period, i.e., splitting it into two or more intervals.

Table 3-8. Development of Myocardial Infarction in Framingham after 16 Years, Men Age 35 to 44, by Level of Serum Cholesterol

Serum cholesterol (mg %)	Developed MI	Did not develop MI	Total
>250	10	125	135
≤250	21	449	470

Source: D. Shurtleff, *The Framingham Study: An Epidemiologic Investigation of Cardiovascular Disease,* Section 26. Washington, D.C.: U.S. GPO, 1970.

USE OF ODDS RATIO IN SAMPLE SIZE CALCULATIONS

Sample size calculations for retrospective studies use the principles outlined in Chapter 2 for a prospective clinical trial, but some differences are worth noting.

Rarely, if ever, is a retrospective study sample size calculation based on specified alternatives for P, such as P_c and P_e. The investigator is much more likely to calculate the sample size needed to detect a significant difference between cases and controls if the proportion with the suspected risk factor among noncases is P_c and the risk factor is associated with an odds ratio of K or more. As a specific illustration, the investigator may want to know the sample size needed to establish a statistically significant difference between intestinal cancer cases and controls with respect to the proportion who state that they usually eat high-fiber foods fewer than two times per week. This calculation requires an assumption, such as "the proportion of the general public eating high-fiber foods less frequently than two times per week is about 70 percent." An additional requirement for this calculation is the specification by the investigator of what level of risk the sample should have a high probability of detecting. This can be specified as "low-fiber diets are associated with an odds ratio of 2 or more." It is also necessary to specify the type I error and type II error that apply identically to prospective and retrospective studies.

For prospective studies, all the elements needed for sample size calculation are present: α, β, P_c, and P_e, the latter two being the binominal parameters for the groups being compared. For retrospective studies, we have α, β, P_c, and OR (instead of P_e). However, it is a simple matter to use P_c and OR to derive the P_e implied by them. Using the illustration of the relationship of a low-fiber diet to intestinal cancer, we organize the relevant data into a 2×2 table relating to population data (not sample estimates) as follows:

Diet	Cases			Noncases (controls)
Low-fiber diet (high-fiber food less frequently than 2 times per week)	$100P_e$	A	B	70
Not low-fiber diet (high-fiber food at least 2 times per week)	$100(1 - P_e)$	C	D	30
Total	100			100

We have arbitrarily established the table for 100 cases and 100 controls. Any other numbers would serve as well, but 100 is a convenient choice. Since one of the conditions underlying our calculation is that 70 percent of the general public eats a low-fiber diet, and since the general public and noncases of intestinal cancer are almost equivalent, we have designated 70 of the 100 controls as on low-fiber diets. If we now put $100P_e$ (100 times the proportion of cases reporting a low-fiber diet) into cell A and $100(1 - P_e)$ into cell C, we transform the proportions into numbers totalling 100 cases and have completed the 2×2 table. The remaining condition to be used is that the specified odds ratio, i.e., the odds ratio we wish to be able to detect if it is true, is

$$OR = \frac{AD}{BC} = 2$$

Using the data in the table, we can now write

$$\frac{AD}{BC} = \frac{100\,P_e\,(30)}{70\,(100)\,(1 - P_e)} = 2$$

Solving for P_e, we obtain $P_e = .82$

If we specify α and β as .05 and .10, respectively, we have all the ingredients for sample size calculation for a retrospective study and can apply the formulas in Chapter 1.

$$P_c = .70 \qquad \alpha = .05$$
$$P_e = .82 \qquad \beta = .10$$

It is probably not at all obvious that if 70 percent of controls and 82 percent of cases eat a low-fiber diet the odds ratio associated with these data is 2. This is precisely why retrospective studies do not formulate their sample size queries using P_c and P_e but use P_c and OR instead. For the reader who is curious, I have calculated sample size for this illustrative retrospective study using Equation 2-

Table 3-9. Sample Size Requirements for Prospective and Retrospective Studies*

Disease incidence in unexposed group	Frequency of attribute in population (%)	Detectable relative risk	Sample size needed in each group	
			Prospective	Retrospective
1/1000	50	1.2	576 732	2535
		2.0	31 443	177
		4.0	5 815	48
1/100	50	1.2	57 100	2535
		2.0	3 100	177
		4.0	567	48
1/10	50	1.2	5 137	2535
		2.0	266	177
		4.0	42	48

* Two-sided $\alpha = .05$; $\beta = .10$.
Source: J. Tonascia, unpublished notes.

6 and found that 288 cases and 288 controls are the numbers required. Good discussions of sample size requirements contrasting prospective and retrospective studies, together with convenient reference tables, can be found in works by Schlesselman [29,30] and Walter [31]. Retrospective studies generally require many fewer cases than prospective ones to investigate equivalent problems, as illustrated in Table 3-9. This is so because it is not necessary to have as many individuals without disease (for comparison to the cases) as are generated in prospective studies of disease with low or moderate incidence.

NOTE

* Some prefer the term *case-control studies*. I am satisfied with either term and use them interchangeably.

4

Attributable Risk

If you "know" that activity A multiplies the risk of lung cancer by 10 and that activity B multiplies the risk of lung cancer by 20 (i.e., $\hat{RR}_A = 10$ and $\hat{RR}_B = 20$), is it correct to infer (assuming very narrow confidence limits on both RR_A and RR_B) that activity B has a greater effect on the public than activity A? Assuming that a county health department has resources to reduce or eliminate one of these hazards but not both, is an attack on B potentially of greater benefit than one on A? Suppose A were cigarette smoking and B were uranium mining and 40 percent of the adults in the county smoke cigarettes but only 0.04 percent mine uranium. Although those who mine uranium are at very great relative risk, the effect of this high risk on the community is small because few individuals are exposed to the risk factor. Clearly the effect of a risk factor on community health is related to both relative risk and the percentage of population exposed to the factor.

Attributable risk is an epidemiologic concept combining relative risk and risk factor prevalence so as to reflect the fraction of all cases associated with the risk factor. As a first step in developing a formula for attributable risk, the following terms are defined:

I_0 incidence rate among those not exposed to the risk factor
I_r incidence rate among those exposed to the risk factor
RR relative risk I_r/I_0
P proportion of the population exposed to the risk factor
N size of the population

Then $I_r - I_0$ is the excess incidence rate among those exposed to the risk factor and $(I_r - I_0)/I_r$ is that proportion of the incidence rate among those with the risk factor due to association with the risk factor. Dividing each term in this proportion by I_0, we can express that proportion of the incidence rate *among those with the risk factor* "due to" association with the risk factor as

$$\left(\frac{I_r}{I_0} - \frac{I_0}{I_0}\right) \bigg/ \frac{I_r}{I_0} = \frac{RR - 1}{RR} \qquad \text{provided } RR \geqslant 1 \qquad (4\text{-}1)$$

The incidence rate due to the risk factor *among those with the factor* is then

$$I_r\left(\frac{RR - 1}{RR}\right) \qquad \text{provided } RR \geqslant 1$$

The number of cases due to association with the risk factor is the term above multiplied by the number in the population having the risk factor (NP):

$$NPI_r\left(\frac{RR - 1}{RR}\right) \qquad \text{provided } RR \geqslant 1$$

where NPI_r is the total number of cases occurring among those with the risk factor.

Thus the attributable risk, which is the number of cases due to association with the risk factor divided by total cases in the population (or the proportion of total cases due to the risk factor) is

$$AR = \frac{NPI_r\left(\dfrac{RR - 1}{RR}\right)}{NPI_r + N(1 - P)I_0} \qquad \text{provided } RR \geqslant 1 \qquad (4\text{-}2)$$

where $N(1 - P)I_0$ is the total number of cases occurring among those without the risk factor.

Dividing each term in Equation 4-2 by NI_0 and simplifying, we get an expression for attributable risk as originally reported by Levin [32]:

$$AR = \frac{P(RR)\left(\dfrac{RR - 1}{RR}\right)}{P(RR) + (1 - P)} = \frac{P(RR - 1)}{1 + P(RR - 1)} \qquad \text{provided } RR \geqslant 1$$

$$(4\text{-}3)$$

In actual practice we substitute $\hat{RR}$ and p for RR and P, respectively, in Equation 4-3:

$$\hat{AR} = \frac{p(\hat{RR} - 1)}{1 + p(\hat{RR} - 1)} \qquad \text{provided } \hat{RR} \geqslant 1 \qquad (4\text{-}4)$$

When the relative risk (or odds ratio) is very high, it strongly suggests that the association so identified is real [33] rather than something spurious derived from various confounding factors (Chapter 5). When the attributable risk is high (the range is from 0 to 1), the risk factor is of importance to the health of the community. Table 4-1 shows some examples of the relationship between RR and AR with respect to risk factors and coronary heart disease among Framingham men [28].

Although Equation 4-3 requires RR for its calculation, the odds ratio may be used as a substitute if the disease is rare in the population.

Attributable risk, as given in Equation 4-3 and as generally used, is a relative measure relating to the total population. However, attributable risk could be expressed in absolute rather than relative terms, that is, in terms of the *total number of cases* due to the risk factor, which in our notation is $NPI_r [(RR − 1)/RR]$. It also might be expressed as a relative measure relating only to those exposed to the risk factor; this is $(RR − 1)/RR$, as stated in Equation 4-1. Other terms that have been used for attributable risk are attributable fraction [34], population attributable risk [35], and aetiologic fraction [36].

Formulas for $\text{vâr}(AR)$ are most easily expressed in notation corresponding to the standard notation we have used for the 2×2 table and which we repeat in Table 4-2. Note that the symbols in Table 4-2 are not specific for prospective or retrospective studies. Thus for a prospective study based on a sample of the general population in which "disease $+$" represents incident cases, (and which is of sufficiently short duration that the dates on which cases occurred can be

Table 4-1. Association of Relative Risk and Attributable Risk for Coronary Heart Disease Among Framingham Men Age 35 to 44 on Initial Examination

Risk factor at initial examination	$R\hat{R}$ at 16-year follow-up*	Proportion of population studied with risk factor at initial examination (p)	$A\hat{R}$ using Equation 4-4	Comment
Systolic blood pressure ≥ 180	2.8	.02	.03	Uncommon risk factors will rarely lead to a high $A\hat{R}$
Enlarged heart on X-ray	2.1	.10	.10	Compared to cigarette smoking, $R\hat{R}$ somewhat higher but $A\hat{R}$ much lower
Cigarette smoking	1.9	.72	.39	Lowest $R\hat{R}$ in table, but almost 40% of all coronary disease is associated with cigarettes

* Relative to those without the risk factor.
Source: D. Shurtleff, *The Framingham Study: An Epidemiologic Investigation of Cardiovascular Disease*, Section 26. Washington, D.C.: U.S. GPO, 1970.

Table 4-2. Notation for Cross-Classification of Disease
and Risk Factor

Risk factor	Disease		Total
	+	−	
+	a	b	$a + b$
−	c	d	$c + d$
Total	$a + c$	$b + d$	t

ignored), the proportion with the risk factor can usually be estimated by $(a + b)/t$. For retrospective studies in which 'disease −" refers to controls representing the general population, the proportion with the risk factor can be estimated by $b/(b + d)$. Also, for prospective data arranged as in Table 4-2, $\hat{RR}$ is derived from $a/(a + b) \div c/(c + d)$. For retrospective data, the relative risk would be estimated, when appropriate, by ad/bc, the odds ratio. Thus, using the notation in Table 4-2, we require two separate formulas for $\hat{var}(AR)$ [37]:

$$\hat{var}(AR) \text{ for prospective data } = \frac{ct[ad(t - c) + bc^2]}{(a + c)^3(c + d)^3} \tag{4-5}$$

$$\hat{var}(AR) \text{ for retrospective data } = \left[\frac{c(b + d)}{d(a + c)}\right]^2 \left[\frac{a}{c(a + c)} + \frac{b}{d(b + d)}\right] \tag{4-6}$$

To illustrate the calculations, we shall use Equations 4-4 and 4-5 in conjunction with data from a large prospective study of smoking and mortality to estimate 95 percent confidence limits on AR for lung cancer related to smoking cigarettes. The data are shown in Table 4-3.

First we calculate $\hat{RR}$ and p from Table 4-3 to estimate RR and P, respectively. As these are prospective data, $\hat{RR} = (1116/701\,768) \div (382/975\,392) = 4.06$ and $p = 701\,768/1\,677\,160 = .42$. The $\hat{RR}$ of 4.06 is much lower than usually quoted for the relationship between cigarette smoking and lung cancer. Most calculations of this $\hat{RR}$ relate the risk among current cigarette smokers to the risk among those who have never smoked. However, the present calculation relates the risk among current cigarette smokers, including light smokers, to the risk among all others, including ex-smokers, pipe smokers, and cigar smokers. When the population is dichotomized, the $\hat{RR}$ refers to the ratio of risk among those with the factor to risk among those without it and the prevalence of the risk factor (p) refers to prevalence in the total population. When two population groups that do not encompass the entire population are contrasted, as, for example, those who are heavy cigarette smokers and those who have never smoked, the $\hat{RR}$ resulting from this more extreme comparison can be used in the formula for $\hat{AR}$, but the

Table 4-3. Current Cigarette Smoking and Mortality Among U.S. Veterans

Smoking category	Lung cancer mortality		Total population
	+	−	
Current cigarette smokers	1116 (a)	700 652 (b)	701 768 $(a + b)$
All others	382 (c)	975 010 (d)	975 392 $(c + d)$
Total	1498 $(a + c)$	1 675 662 $(b + d)$	1 677 160 (t)

Note: person-years of observation in the original report are considered here, and in the text, as if they were separate individuals.
Source: H. A. Kahn, National Cancer Institute Monograph 19, (1966).

risk factor prevalence used with it must be that appropriate to just the two categories being considered. These calculations can be based on the Table 4-2 format if "risk factor +" and "risk factor −" define the restricted categories. The attributable risk resulting from a nonexhaustive two-category comparison should be understood as the fraction of *the cases in the two limited categories* associated with the high risk factor.

In addition, if the reference category is one such as "never smoked," the cases attributed to smoking would have to be understood as cases in excess of the rate observed for those who had never smoked. Conceptually this excess could be completely eliminated only by converting the population to one that never smoked and not just to a population of ex-smokers.

Inserting the previously calculated values of $\hat{RR}$ and p into Equation 4-4, we get

$$\hat{AR} = \frac{.42(3.06)}{1 + .42(3.06)} = .56$$

Thus we estimate that 56 percent of the lung cancer that occurs in the population under consideration is associated with current cigarette smoking. Since this calculation derived from dichotomizing the complete population data, it is at least imaginable that, if the cigarette smoking–lung cancer association is casual, 56 percent of lung cancer mortality could be eliminated by converting the population from current cigarette smokers to ex-smokers or to pipe or cigar smokers.

To calculate $\hat{var}(AR)$ for a prospective study, we substitute the data of Table 4-3 (which follows the format of Table 4-2) into Equation 4-5:

$$\hat{var}\,AR = \frac{382(1\,677\,160)[1116(975\,010)(1\,677\,160 - 382) + 700\,652(382)^2]}{(1116 + 382)^3(382 + 975\,010)^3}$$

$$= .000\,375$$

$$\hat{SE}(AR) = (.000375)^{1/2} = .019$$

$$1.96\ \hat{SE}(AR) = .038$$

Thus on the basis of this large data set we calculate the 95 percent confidence limits on AR as .56 ± .04, or .52 to .60.

To illustrate the use of the retrospective formula for vâr (AR), imagine that we have been able to identify all the lung cancer deaths in Table 4-3 as well as a perfectly representative one per 1000 sample of the rest as controls. These data, which are shown in Table 4-4, are essentially identical to the data of Table 4-3 except for the great reduction in the number of those not dying of lung cancer. The point of this illustration is to show how the variance of $\hat{AR}$ changes between prospective and retrospective studies with equivalent relationships. From Table 4-4

$$\hat{RR} \cong \hat{OR} = \frac{1116(975)}{701(382)} = 4.06$$

$$p = \frac{701}{1676} = .42$$

$$\hat{AR} = \frac{p(\hat{RR}-1)}{1+p(\hat{RR}-1)} = \frac{.42(3.06)}{1 + .42(3.06)} = .56$$

Using Equation 4-6,

$$\sqrt{\text{vâr}(AR)} \text{ retrospective} = \left\{\left[\frac{382(1676)}{975(1498)}\right]^2 \left[\frac{1116}{382(1498)} + \frac{701}{975(1676)}\right]\right\}^{1/2}$$

$$= .0214$$

$$1.96\sqrt{\text{vâr}(AR)} = .042$$

Thus using Tables 4-3 and 4-4 for basic data sources, our comparison is as follows:

	Prospective	Retrospective
$\hat{RR}$	4.06	4.06
p	.42	.42
$\hat{AR}$	.56	.56
95% CL on AR	.522 and .598	.518 and .602

Table 4-4. Retrospective Data Derived from Table 4-3

Smoking category	Lung cancer mortality		Total
	+	−	
Current cigarette smokers	1116 (a)	701 (b)	1817
All others	382 (c)	975 (d)	1457
Total	1498 $(a + c)$	1676 $(b + d)$	3174

The only difference relates to the slightly wider confidence limits computed from the very much smaller (although still quite large) sample size of the retrospective study.

The definition and measurement of attributable risk may be approached in a different way. Suppose 40 percent of all *cases* are in the high-risk category and the proportion of the high-risk incidence rate due to the risk factor, $(I_r - I_0)/I_r$, is 60 percent. Then .40(.60), or 24 percent, of all cases are attributable to the high-risk factor. More generally, using Equation 4-1 and the notation of Table 4-2, this formulation of $\hat{AR}$ can be expressed as

$$\hat{AR} = \left(\frac{a}{a + c}\right)\left(\frac{\hat{RR} - 1}{\hat{RR}}\right) \qquad \text{provided } \hat{RR} \geqslant 1. \qquad (4\text{-}7)$$

Equation 4-7 can be recognized as the basis of Equation 4-8, which calculates attributable risk after adjustment for confounding factors by means of the standardized morbidity ratio (SMR) [36]. The summation in Equation 4-8 is over each category of the confounding variable(s):

$$\hat{AR} = \sum_i \left(\frac{a_i}{a_i + c_i}\right)\left(\frac{\hat{SMR}_i - 1}{\hat{SMR}_i}\right) \qquad \text{provided each } \hat{SMR}_i \geqslant 1 \qquad (4\text{-}8)$$

Several times in our discussion we have referred to disease "due to" association with the risk factor. In fact, all the calculations of attributable risk summarize the proportion of disease *associated with* a risk factor. Whether the disease is caused by the risk factor must be determined on other criteria, as outlined in basic texts on epidemiology [8, 17–19]. Direct experimentation to discover whether eliminating the risk factor eliminates the disease associated with it is usually difficult and expensive and is rarely undertaken. More commonly, indirect indicators are relied upon to suggest whether or not a change in risk factor level has resulted in a change in risk.

5

Adjustment of Data Without Use of Multivariate Models

Often, in analyzing epidemiologic data, the investigator wishes to adjust for the effect of some variable so that the effect of other variables can be seen more clearly. Consider the simple example of an investigation to determine whether or not gray hair is related to mortality risk. The following two facts stand out:

1. Those with gray hair have a higher death rate than others.
2. Those with gray hair are older than others.

Because of fact 2, the interpretation of fact 1 is unclear. The possible association of gray hair with mortality risk is entangled with the effect of age on mortality risk. Methods for adjusting data to overcome this entanglement are among the common tools used by epidemiologists. The purpose of data adjustment is to disentangle the relationship so that we can evaluate a variable's effect free from confusion and distortion. For the gray hair investigation, adjustment would permit us to determine whether *persons of the same age* who have or do not have gray hair have different mortality risks.

CONFOUNDING

Variables whose effect is entangled with the effect of other variables are known as *confounders*, and it is for such variables that data adjustment is needed. In order for a variable to be a confounder, it must be related to the disease or condition of interest *and* to the risk factor being investigated [38]. Stated more exactly, it must be related to the disease or condition of interest *and* to the risk factor being investigated after adjustment for all other risk factors under consideration [39].

A very common application of adjustment to remove confounding is the age adjustment of mortality rates. This permits comparison of mortality risk for various groups free from the distortion introduced by one group having a different age distribution than another. Our first example of confounding uses vital statistics rates, wherein the condition of interest is the death rate and the risk factor to be evaluated is geographic area. When age is associated with area, i.e., the population of one area is much younger (or older) than another, the association of area with mortality risk is confounded by the association of age with mortality risk. If areas differ, as they probably do, in the proportion of the population reading two or more books a year, adjustment of mortality rates to eliminate confounding with this literary variable is unnecessary since reading is (presumably) not related to mortality risk.

We shall discuss two types of age adjustment in relation to mortality rates: direct adjustment and indirect adjustment. The following notation is for sample data and is applicable to both methods:

a	area a
b	area b
s	area chosen as a reference standard
n_{ia}	number of individuals in ith age class of area a
n_{ib}	number of individuals in ith age class of area b
n_{is}	number of individuals in ith age class of standard area
x_{ia}	number of deaths in ith age class of area a (similarly for b and s)
$p_{ia} = \dfrac{x_{ia}}{n_{ia}}$	death rate in ith age class of area a (similarly for b and s)

DIRECT ADJUSTMENT

The basic idea of direct adjustment, or direct standardization, is to suppose that both area a and area b have the age distribution of the standard area instead of the age distributions they actually have. Standardized rates are then calculated for each area, making use of the standard age distribution. These adjusted rates are then compared, and any difference between them can no longer be due to difference in age distribution because age has been taken into account.

The estimated mortality rates for areas a and b calculated by the direct method are

$$D\hat{S}R_a = \text{directly standardized mortality rate for area a}$$

$$= \frac{\sum\limits_{i} p_{ia} n_{is}}{\sum\limits_{i} n_{is}} \tag{5-1}$$

$$D\hat{S}R_b = \text{directly standardized mortality rate for area b}$$

$$= \frac{\sum\limits_{i} p_{ib} n_{is}}{\sum\limits_{i} n_{is}} \tag{5-2}$$

Since $\sum\limits_{i} n_{is}$ is a constant, these equations can also be written in the form

$$D\hat{S}R_a = \sum_i p_{ia}\left(\frac{n_{is}}{\sum\limits_i n_{is}}\right)$$

$$D\hat{S}R_b = \sum_i p_{ib}\left(\frac{n_{is}}{\sum\limits_i n_{is}}\right) \tag{5-3}$$

Thus in each area the age-specific mortality rate for the ith age group has been multiplied by $(n_{is}/\sum\limits_i n_{is})$ and the product then summed over all ages. This is equivalent to obtaining a weighted combination of the age-specific mortality rates using *exactly the same weighting factors* in each area.

If a different standard population had been chosen, a different weighting of age-specific rates would have resulted. Much has been written about the choice of standard populations, emphasizing that in extreme cases the choice of different standard populations can lead to different results. It is even possible that with one standard population the standardized mortality rate for area a will be larger than for area b and with another standard population the standardized mortality rate for b will be larger than for a. The following factors should be considered in choosing a standard population:

1. Select a population that is relevant to the data.
2. Within wide ranges of choice, the population chosen as a standard usually does not make much difference.
3. Understand fully what you are doing in calculating directly standardized rates. If the age-specific rates for area a are greater than for area b at young ages and the opposite is true at older ages, a population giving more weight to younger than to older ages will result in the directly standardized rate for area a exceeding that for area b. A population giving more weight to older than to younger ages will have the opposite result. Obviously the combining of age-specific data into a standardized overall rate is a convenience. However, do not forget that the age-specific data are the "facts" and that their combination into a weighted average, while often useful, is simply an attempt to summarize these facts into one index.

Since the choice of a particular standard population is somewhat arbitrary, I suggest considering, when two areas are to be standardized, a standard population that relates to the variance of the difference between standardized rates for areas a and b. For each age-specific comparison $p_{ia} - p_{ib}$, the variance of the difference is proportional to

$$\frac{1}{n_{ia}} + \frac{1}{n_{ib}}$$

By using the *inverse* of this quantity,

$$\frac{1}{\dfrac{1}{n_{ia}} + \dfrac{1}{n_{ib}}} = \frac{n_{ia}n_{ib}}{n_{ia} + n_{ib}}$$

as a population size or weighting factor for the ith age class, we tend to give more weight to age-specific comparisons with small sampling variance and less weight to age-specific comparisons with large sampling variance.

Common choices for a standard population include total population of the groups to be compared, the population of one of the groups in the comparison, a large population (such as that of the United States), and weighting factors inversely proportional to the variance of the difference between areas. The last is useful when only two groups are being compared. If several groups are being standardized, the variance of the difference between p_{ia} and p_{ib} relates to n_{ia} and n_{ib} and the variance of the difference between p_{ia} and p_{ic} necessarily involves n_{ia} and n_{ic}. Thus weighting factors inversely proportional to the variance of the difference will vary depending on the specific groups being compared, and such factors become impractical for direct standardization of more than two areas.

To illustrate direct standardization methods with a specific example, we use the data in Tables 5-1 and 5-2 on 1970 mortality rates in California and Maine [40, 41] to compare mortality risk in these two states. In what follows, we shall use the symbol w_i to represent $n_{is}/\sum_i n_{is}$ or any alternative form of the standard population in the ith age class.

Table 5-1. 1970 Mortality Data to Illustrate Direct and Indirect Adjustment

Age (i)	United states (standard population s) Pop. in thousands ($n_{is}/1000$)	Number of deaths (x_{is})	California (a) Pop. in thousands ($n_{ia}/1000$)	Number of deaths (x_{ia})	Maine (b) Pop. in thousands ($n_{ib}/1000$)	Number of deaths (x_{ib})
<15	57 900	103 062	5 524	8 751	286	535
15–24	35 441	45 261	3 558	4 747	168	192
25–34	24 907	39 193	2 677	4 036	110	152
35–44	23 088	72 617	2 359	6 701	109	313
45–54	23 220	169 517	2 330	15 675	110	759
55–64	18 590	308 373	1 704	26 276	94	1 622
65–74	12 436	445 531	1 105	36 259	69	2 690
75+	7 630	736 758	696	63 840	46	4 788
Total (excluding unknown ages)	203 212	1 920 312	19 953	166 285	992	11 051

Source: *Characteristics of the Population*, vol. 1, part I, U.S. Summary section I; Washington, D.C.: U.S. Bureau of the Census, 1970; and *Vital Statistics of the U.S.*, vol. II, part B; Washington, D.C.: National Center for Health Statistics, 1970.

Table 5-2. Summary Statistics Derived from Table 5-1

| Age (i) | Weights for direct standardization | | Age-specific rate[a] | | | Under the null hypothesis | |
	Based on standard population $\left(w_i = \dfrac{n_{is}}{\sum_i n_{is}}\right)$	Inversely proportional to variance of $p_{ia} - p_{ib}$ $\left[w_i = \dfrac{1}{\left(\dfrac{1}{n_{ia}} + \dfrac{1}{n_{ib}}\right)} = \dfrac{n_{ia}n_{ib}}{n_{ia}+n_{ib}}\right]$	U.S. (p_{is})	California (p_{ia})	Maine (p_{ib})	Pooled rate for Maine and California[a] $\left(p_i = \dfrac{n_{ia}p_{ia}+n_{ib}p_{ib}}{n_{ia}+n_{ib}}\right)$	Estimated variance within age classes $(p_i q_i)$
<15	.285	272 000	1.8	1.6	1.9	1.6	.0016
15–24	.174	160 000	1.3	1.3	1.1	1.3	.0013
25–34	.123	106 000	1.6	1.5	1.4	1.5	.0015
35–44	.114	104 000	3.1	2.8	2.9	2.8	.0028
45–54	.114	105 000	7.3	6.7	6.9	6.7	.0067
55–64	.091	89 000	16.6	15.4	17.3	15.5	.0153
65–74	.061	65 000	35.8	32.8	39.0	33.2	.0321
75+	.038	43 000	96.6	91.7	104.1	92.5	.0839
Total	1.000	944 000	—	—	—	—	—
Crude rates	—	—	9.4	8.3	11.1	—	—

[a] All rates are per 1000 population.

In Table 5-2 the standard weighting factors based on the U.S. population are calculated as the proportion that each age class in the standard is to the total, e.g., for under age 15, $w_{<15} = 57\,900/203\,212 = .285$. The standard weighting factors that are inversely proportional to the variance of the difference between p_{ia} and p_{ib} are the product of n_{ia} and n_{ib} divided by their sum. For example, for age < 15,

$$w_{<15} = \frac{5\,524\,000\,(286\,000)}{5\,524\,000 + 286\,000} \cong 272\,000$$

Note that in this instance we use the full sample size in each state rather than $n_i/1000$. For directly standardized weighting factors, it was immaterial. Dividing numerator and denominator by 1000 does not affect w_i. For "inverse variance" weighting factors, however, using the actual sample size rather than the sample size in thousands does affect w_i. It increases it 1000-fold. Multiplying each w_i by 1000 does not affect $D\hat{S}R$, but it does affect $\hat{var}(DSR)$. Perhaps the first thing to note in Table 5-2 is that, without adjustment for age, the mortality rate for Maine is higher than for California:

Crude rate per 1000 for California (a)   8.3
Crude rate per 1000 for Maine (b)   11.1
Relative risk (Maine/California)   11.1/8.3 = 1.34

Direct adjustment (as in Equation 5-3) using the U.S. population for standard weighting factors results in

$D\hat{S}R_a = 8.8$ per 1000 (using standard population weighting factors)

$D\hat{S}R_b = 9.9$ per 1000 (using standard population weighting factors)

Note that removing the confounding effect of age reduces the relative risk (Maine/California) from 1.34 to 9.9/8.8 = 1.12.

If instead of using standard population weighting factors in Equation 5-3 we use factors inversely proportional to the variance of $p_{ia} - p_{ib}$, we would have

$D\hat{S}R_a = 9.8$ per 1000 (using weighting factors inversely proportional to variance)

$D\hat{S}R_b = 11.0$ per 1000 (using weighting factors inversely proportional to variance)

With these weighting factors, the relative risk (Maine/California) is 11.0/9.8 = 1.12, unchanged from that obtained using the standard population as a source of constant weighting factors. It is interesting to observe that, when the different standards are used, the adjusted rates do differ but their ratio remains the same. Of course, a mortality rate that has been standardized by the direct method is not meaningful by itself; it has meaning only when compared with another mortality rate that has been similarly standardized.

Variance of the Difference Between Directly Standardized Rates

We begin by recalling three rules related to the calculation of variances (Equations 1-9, 1-10, and 1-17):

1. The variance of the difference between independent variables is the sum of their variances: $\text{var}(x - y) = \text{var}(x) + \text{var}(y)$.
2. The variance of a variable multiplied by a constant is the variance of the variable multiplied by the constant squared: $\text{var}(Kx) = K^2 \text{var}(x)$.
3. The estimated variances of p_{ia} and p_{ib} are $p_i q_i / n_{ia}$ and $p_i q_i / n_{ib}$, respectively, where p_i is the estimate of the parameter under the null hypothesis and is computed as the weighted average of p_{ia} and p_{ib}:

$$p_i = \frac{n_{ia} p_{ia} + n_{ib} p_{ib}}{n_{ia} + n_{ib}}$$

We shall use these rules to calculate the variance of the difference between two directly standardized rates.

We want $\text{vâr}(DSR_a - DSR_b)$, which, using Equation 5-3, can be written

$$\text{vâr} \left(\frac{\sum_i p_{ia} w_i}{\sum_i w_i} - \frac{\sum_i p_{ib} w_i}{\sum_i w_i} \right)$$

with each term divided by $\sum w_i$ to cover instances wherein $\sum w_i \neq 1$. Applying Equations 1-9, 1-10, and 1-17,

$$\text{vâr}(DSR_a - DSR_b) = \frac{\sum_i p_i q_i w_i^2}{\left(\sum_i w_i\right)^2 n_{ia}} + \frac{\sum_i p_i q_i w_i^2}{\left(\sum_i w_i\right)^2 n_{ib}}$$

which can be written

$$\text{vâr}(DSR_a - DSR_b) = \frac{\sum_i p_i q_i w_i^2}{\left(\sum_i w_i\right)^2} \left(\frac{1}{n_{ia}} + \frac{1}{n_{ib}}\right) \qquad (5\text{-}4)$$

If we are using weighting factors inversely proportional to the variance of $p_{ia} - p_{ib}$, however, then

$$\frac{1}{n_{ia}} + \frac{1}{n_{ib}} = \frac{1}{w_i}$$

and

$$\hat{var}(DSR_a - DSR_b) = \frac{\sum_i p_i q_i w_i^2}{\left(\sum_i w_i\right)^2}\left(\frac{1}{w_i}\right)$$

so that

$$\hat{var}(DSR_a - DSR_b) = \frac{\sum_i p_i q_i w_i}{\left(\sum_i w_i\right)^2} \qquad (5\text{-}5)$$

If inverse variance weighting factors are not used, then the simplification embodied in Equation 5-5 does not apply. Whatever the choice of weighting factors the variance of the difference between directly standardized rates can be estimated by Equation 5-4.

Using Equation 5-4 for the variance of the difference between the adjusted rates for California and Maine based on *standard* population weighting factors we have

$$\hat{var}(DSR_a - DSR_b) = \frac{\sum_i p_i q_i w_i^2}{\left(\sum_i w_i\right)^2}\left(\frac{1}{n_{ia}} + \frac{1}{n_{ib}}\right)$$

If $\sum_i w_i = 1$, this becomes

$$\sum_i p_i q_i w_i^2\left(\frac{1}{n_{ia}} + \frac{1}{n_{ib}}\right)$$

Substituting Table 5-2 data beginning with age class under 15 and age class 15 to 24 leads to

$$.0016(.285)^2\left(\frac{1}{272\,000}\right) + .0013(.174)^2\left(\frac{1}{160\,000}\right) + \ldots$$

Note: in Table 5-2, the column "Weights inversely proportional to variance . . ." shows

$$\frac{1}{\dfrac{1}{n_{ia}} + \dfrac{1}{n_{ib}}}$$

The reciprocal of that quantity provides $(1/n_{ia}) + (1/n_{ib})$, as wanted for Equation 5-4.

Completing this summation over all age classes leads to

$$\hat{var}(DSR_a - DSR_b) = .000000008196$$

$$\hat{SE}(DSR_a - DSR_b) = .000091$$

(for standard population weighting factors). Remember that $D\hat{S}R$ values have been written as "per thousand", thus a $D\hat{S}R_a$ value of 8.8/1000 actually equals .0088 and a $D\hat{S}R_b$ value of 9.9/1000 = .0099. Their difference, .0088 − .0099 = − .0011, when divided by the standard error of the difference, which is .000091, permits a test of the null hypothesis that this difference is simply a chance departure from zero. For this test we use

$$z = \frac{\text{difference} - \text{expected value of difference under H}_0}{\hat{SE} \text{ of difference}} = \frac{-.0011 - 0}{.000091}$$

$$= -12$$

This z value is far beyond the limits of chance fluctuation and suggests a differential mortality risk between Maine and California, apart from any differences in age structure of the two populations.

Using Equation 5-5 to calculate the variance of the difference between California and Maine adjusted rates based on weighting factors inversely proportional to the variance of $p_{ia} - p_{ib}$, we have

$$\hat{var}(DSR_a - DSR_b) = \sum_i p_i q_i w_i \bigg/ \left(\sum_i w_i \right)^2 = [.0016(272\,000)$$

$$+ .0013(160\,000) + \ldots]/(944\,000)^2$$

$$\hat{var}(DSR_a - DSR_b) = .000000009934$$

$$\hat{SE}(DSR_a - DSR_b) = .000100$$

Again shifting from rate per 1000 to straight proportions, $DSR_a - DSR_b$ for inverse variance weighting factors is .0098 − .0110 = − .0012 and the test of the null hypothesis that both areas have the same risk with observed differences simply due to chance fluctuation is

$$z = \frac{-.0012 - 0}{.000100} = -12$$

as before. Thus both sets of weighting factors lead to the same conclusion: Maine has a higher mortality risk than California, after adjusting for age.

It should be noted that large data sets such as these almost always show significant differences. Keep in mind that *significance* (which is equivalent to *unusualness*) depends on the difference in relation to its standard error and that the latter depends on *sample size*. For very large samples, even the most trivial differences will be statistically significant.

INDIRECT ADJUSTMENT

Sometimes direct adjustment, or standardization, cannot be carried out because the age-specific rates in the groups to be standardized are not available or, in at least some age classes, are based on such small numbers as to be completely unreliable. Indirect standardization does not require area age-specific rates but does require

1. Age distribution of each group to be standardized
2. Total deaths in each group to be standardized
3. Age-specific rates for a standard population

The indirect method uses items 1 and 3 to calculate how many deaths would be expected in each group if the age-specific rates of the standard population were applicable. This expectation is then compared with the actual number of deaths in the group. This observed/expected ratio is a relative, indirect, age-adjusted rate and is (after multiplication by 100) frequently referred to as a standardized mortality ratio (*SMR*). By using the notation defined at the beginning of this chapter, we shall see how *SMR* is related to the indirectly standardized rate (*ISR*):

$$\frac{\sum_i p_{is} n_{ia}}{\sum_i n_{ia}} = \text{crude rate in area a if age-specific rates of the standard population are applied}$$

$$\frac{\sum_i p_{is} n_{is}}{\sum_i n_{is}} = \text{crude rate in standard population}$$

The ratio of the crude rate in the standard population to the crude rate in area a if age-specific rates of the standard population are applied is

$$\frac{\sum_i p_{is} n_{is}}{\sum_i n_{is}} \left(\frac{\sum_i n_{ia}}{\sum_i p_{is} n_{ia}} \right) = \text{standardizing factor}$$

Note how this standardizing factor, which varies from group to group only because of differences in age distribution, adjusts for differences in age distribution. If the population of area a is very much older than the standard population, so that using *the same age-specific rates* as the standard the crude rate for area a is double the crude rate for the standard, then the standardizing factor will be $\frac{1}{2}$. Similarly, if the population of area a is much younger than the standard, so that using the *same age-specific rates* as the standard the crude rate for area a is one half that for the standard, then the standardizing factor will be 2. Thus the age distribution is evaluated in relation to the standard, and the standardizing factor increases the crude rate for an area with a population younger than the standard and decreases it for an area with a population older than the standard. The indirect age-adjusted rate is finally the crude rate to be standardized multiplied by the standardizing factor.

$$\text{crude rate} \quad \times \quad \text{standardizing factor}$$

$$\text{Indirect standardized} = \left(\frac{\sum_i p_{ia} n_{ia}}{\sum_i n_{ia}}\right) \left(\frac{\sum_i p_{is} n_{is}}{\sum_i n_{is}} \times \frac{\sum_i n_{ia}}{\sum_i p_{is} n_{ia}}\right) \quad (5\text{-}6)$$

Note that the crude rate for area a has been written in Equation 5-6 as if we had individual age-specific rates, p_{ia}. In fact, we often do not. It is the *sum* of all $p_{ia} n_{ia}$, i.e., the total number of deaths, that we must know.

By cancelling and rearranging terms, Equation 5-6 can be written in the form

$$I\hat{S}R_a = \left(\frac{\sum_i p_{ia} n_{ia}}{\sum_i p_{is} n_{ia}}\right) \left(\frac{\sum_i p_{is} n_{is}}{\sum_i n_{is}}\right) \quad (5\text{-}7)$$

$$= \frac{\text{observed cases in area a}}{\text{expected cases if standard rates applied to population a}} \times \frac{\text{crude rate in}}{\text{standard area}}$$

The *ISR* for area b is identical to that given in Equation 5-7 for area a except that p_{ib} and n_{ib} substitute for p_{ia} and n_{ia}, respectively:

$$I\hat{S}R_b = \left(\frac{\sum_i p_{ib} n_{ib}}{\sum_i p_{is} n_{ib}}\right) \left(\frac{\sum_i p_{is} n_{is}}{\sum_i n_{is}}\right) \quad (5\text{-}8)$$

Comparing $I\hat{S}R_b$ and $I\hat{S}R_a$, we can see that differences relate to the left factor only. In this factor, the numerator is the number of observed deaths in the area being considered and the denominator is the number of deaths expected in that area if standard rates applied. Note that the standard rates are being combined according to the age structure of area b in $I\hat{S}R_b$ and according to the age structure of area a in $I\hat{S}R_a$. Because indirect age-adjusted rates for different areas do not all use exactly the same weighting factors (as would be true for directly adjusted rates), it is technically incorrect to compare $I\hat{S}R_a$ with $I\hat{S}R_b$.

However, $\sum_i p_{ia} n_{ia}$ can always be compared with $\sum_i p_{is} n_{ia}$ and $\sum_i p_{ib} n_{ib}$ can always be compared with $\sum_i p_{is} n_{ib}$ because exactly the same set of weighting factors are used in each element of the comparison. Thus each indirectly adjusted rate is always comparable to the standard. Although, as stated above, it is technically incorrect to compare indirectly adjusted rates for different areas, it is difficult to find practical examples in which such a comparison is a source of substantial error.

The first fraction in Equation 5-7 is the standardized mortality ratio (SMR), which, as stated earlier, is a relative, indirect, age-standardized rate. To convert it to an indirectly standardized rate, simply multiply by the crude rate of the standard population. Recalling that $p_{ia} n_{ia} = x_{ia}$, we can rewrite Equation 5-7 in the form

$$I\hat{S}R_a = \left(\frac{\sum_i x_{ia}}{\sum_i p_{is} n_{ia}} \right) \left(\frac{\sum_i p_{is} n_{is}}{\sum_i n_{is}} \right) \tag{5-9}$$

Variance of Indirectly Adjusted Rates

To estimate the variance of $I\hat{S}R_a$ as shown in Equation 5-9, we shall consider x_{ia} as the only sampling variable since n_{ia} and n_{is} are fixed from sample to sample and p_{is}, which is used for standardization of several areas, can be presumed to be known exactly. Standard rates are frequently based on very large numbers so that even if it is incorrect to regard them as constant from sample to sample, the sampling error is generally very small relative to that for $p_{ia} = x_{ia}/n_{ia}$. Under these conditions, the variance of Equation 5-9 is

$$\text{var}(I\hat{S}R_a) = \frac{\sum_i n_{ia} P_{ia} Q_{ia}}{\left(\sum_i p_{is} n_{ia} \right)^2} \left(\frac{\sum_i p_{is} n_{is}}{\sum_i n_{is}} \right)^2 \tag{5-10}$$

When, as is usual, $p_{ia} q_{ia}$ is substituted for the unknown parameter $P_{ia} Q_{ia}$, we no longer have var$(I\hat{S}R_a)$, but an estimate of it:

$$\hat{\text{var}}(ISR_a) = \frac{\sum_i n_{ia} p_{ia} q_{ia}}{\left(\sum_i p_{is} n_{ia} \right)^2} \left(\frac{\sum_i p_{is} n_{is}}{\sum_i n_{is}} \right)^2 \tag{5-11}$$

The first term on the right-hand side of Equation 5-9 is $S\hat{M}R$, which we have referred to previously. Although it is a component of an indirectly standardized rate, it is also frequently used alone as a method of data adjustment. As can be seen from Equation 5-9, the $S\hat{M}R$ for area a is the ratio of the observed cases in the area divided by the expected cases in the area if the specific rates from the standard population are applied. Since ISR_a is identical to SMR_a except for a constant multiplier, the variances of ISR_a and SMR_a are also identical except for a constant multiplier. Thus, the variance of SMR_a is exactly as Equation 5-11 but omitting the constant multiplier:

$$\left(\frac{\sum_i p_{is} n_{is}}{\sum_i n_{is}}\right)^2$$

which is the square of the crude rate in the standard population, and

$$\text{vâr}(SMR_a) = \frac{\sum_i n_{ia} p_{ia} q_{ia}}{\left(\sum_i p_{is} n_{ia}\right)^2} \qquad (5\text{-}12)$$

If the p_{ia} are small, as they often are, the q_{ia} will be close to unity and

$$\sum_i n_{ia} p_{ia} q_{ia} \cong \sum_i n_{ia} p_{ia} = \sum_i x_{ia}$$

In this event,

$$\text{vâr}(ISR_a) \cong \frac{\sum_i x_{ia}}{\left(\sum_i p_{is} n_{ia}\right)^2} \left(\frac{\sum_i p_{is} n_{is}}{\sum_i n_{is}}\right)^2 \qquad (5\text{-}13)$$

and the estimated variance of SMR_a is approximately

$$\text{vâr}(SMR_a) \cong \frac{\sum_i x_{ia}}{\left(\sum_i p_{is} n_{ia}\right)^2}$$

This is exactly (observed deaths)/(expected deaths)^2, and since (observed deaths)/(expected deaths) $= S\hat{M}R$, the estimated variance of SMR when p_i are small is then

$$\text{vâr}(SMR) \cong \frac{S\hat{M}R}{E} \qquad (5\text{-}14)$$

$$\hat{SE}(SMR) \cong \sqrt{\frac{S\hat{M}R}{E}} \qquad (5\text{-}15)$$

where E is the number of expected deaths. You may also encounter $\hat{SE}(SMR)$ expressed in a different way:

$$\hat{SE}(SMR) \cong \frac{S\hat{M}R}{\sqrt{O}} \tag{5-16}$$

where O is the number of observed deaths. At first glance Equation 5-16 seems to be in disagreement with Equation 5-15, but the exact equivalence of these two equations can be shown as follows. Recall that $SMR = O/E$; then

$$\frac{\sqrt{S\hat{M}R}}{\sqrt{E}} = \frac{\sqrt{\bar{O}}/\sqrt{E}}{\sqrt{E}} \tag{5-15'}$$

$$= \frac{\sqrt{\bar{O}}/\sqrt{E}}{\sqrt{E}} \left(\frac{\sqrt{\bar{O}}/\sqrt{E}}{\sqrt{\bar{O}}/\sqrt{E}} \right)$$

$$= \frac{O/E}{\sqrt{O}} = \frac{S\hat{M}R}{\sqrt{O}} \tag{5-16'}$$

We shall use Tables 5-1 and 5-2 data to illustrate how to calculate Maine and California rates adjusted for age by the indirect method. Remember that for indirect adjustment it is not strictly correct to compare the Maine rate with the California rate. However, each can be properly compared to the standard population. Using Equation 5-9 and U.S. rates for a standard,

$$I\hat{S}R_a = \left(\frac{\sum_i x_{ia}}{\sum_i p_{is} n_{ia}} \right) \left(\frac{\sum_i p_{is} n_{is}}{\sum_i n_{is}} \right)$$

$$= \frac{166\,285}{.0018\,(5\,524\,000) + \ldots .0966\,(696\,000)}\,(.0094)$$

$$= \frac{166\,285}{178\,253}\,(.0094) = .0088$$

Similarly

$$I\hat{S}R_b = \frac{11\,051}{10\,524}\,(.0094) = .0099$$

After indirect adjustment, the California and Maine rates are identical to the rates obtained by direct adjustment using the U.S. population as a standard. Of course, this will not always be true, but differences will usually be slight.

Using Equation 5-11,

$$\text{vâr}(ISR_a) = \frac{5\,524\,000\,(.0016)\,(.9984) + \ldots\ldots 696\,000\,(.0917)\,(.9083)}{(178\,253)^2}\,(.0094)^2$$

$$= \frac{158\,410}{(178\,253)^2}\,(.0094)^2 = .000000000441$$

$$\hat{SE}(ISR_a) = .000021$$

$$\text{vâr}(ISR_b) = \frac{286\,000\,(.0019)\,(.9981) + \ldots 46\,000\,(.1041)\,(.8959)}{(10\,524)^2}\,(.0094)^2$$

$$= \frac{10\,424}{(10\,524)^2}\,(.0094)^2 = .000000008316$$

$$\hat{SE}(ISR_b) = .000091$$

Using the approximation in Equation 5-13 dependent on small p_{ia} and p_{ib},

$$\text{vâr}(ISR_a) \cong \frac{\sum_i x_{ia}}{\left(\sum_i p_{is} n_{ia}\right)^2}\left(\frac{\sum_i p_{is} n_{is}}{\sum_i n_{is}}\right)$$

$$= \frac{166\,285}{(178\,253)^2}\,(.0094)^2 = .000000000462$$

$$\hat{SE}(ISR_a) = .000022$$

$$\text{vâr}(ISR_b) \cong \frac{11\,051}{(10\,524)^2}\,(.0094)^2 = .000000008816$$

$$\hat{SE}(ISR_b) \cong .000094$$

We compare below the standard errors of the indirectly adjusted mortality rates computed by Equations 5-11 and 5-13:

	$\hat{SE}(ISR_a)$	$\hat{SE}(ISR_b)$
Equation 5-11	.000021	.000091
Equation 5-13	.000022	.000094

Note how close the computed standard errors derived from the low p value approximation (Equation 5-13) are to the more accurate estimates (Equation 5-11). This excellent agreement is due to the small p values in our example.

This completes our calculation of indirectly adjusted rates and their standard error based on data in Tables 5-1 and 5-2. The SMR is an element of the indirectly standardized rate, and we now compute these ratios and their standard error. Using the first term in Equations 5-7 and 5-8, we get

$$S\hat{M}R_a = \frac{\sum_i p_{ia} n_{ia}}{\sum_i p_{is} n_{ia}} = \frac{166\,285}{178\,253} = 0.933$$

$$S\hat{M}R_b = \frac{\sum_i p_{ib} n_{ib}}{\sum_i p_{is} n_{ib}} = \frac{11\,051}{10\,524} = 1.050$$

The estimated variance of SMR is obtained from Equation 5-12 or, under the small p_i approximation, from Equation 5-14:

$$\text{vâr}(SMR_a) \text{ using Equation 5-12} = \frac{\sum_i n_{ia} p_{ia} q_{ia}}{\left(\sum_i p_{is} n_{ia}\right)^2} = \frac{158\,410}{(178\,253)^2} = .000004986$$

$$\text{vâr}(SMR_a) \text{ using Equation 5-14} = \frac{S\hat{M}R_a}{E} = \frac{S\hat{M}R_a}{\sum_i p_{is} n_{ia}} = \frac{.93}{178\,253}$$
$$= .000005217$$

$$\text{vâr}(SMR_b) \text{ using Equation 5-12} = \frac{10\,424}{(10\,524)^2} = .000094118$$

$$\text{vâr}(SMR_b) \text{ using Equation 5-14} = \frac{1.05}{10\,524} = .000099772$$

Taking the square roots of these variances, we compare the standard errors of SMR obtained by the two formulas and see that they are very similar:

	$\hat{SE}(SMR_a)$	$\hat{SE}(SMR_b)$
Equation 5-12	.0022	.0097
Equation 5-14	.0023	.0100

We previously stated that it is technically incorrect to compare the indirectly adjusted rates for two areas. The same limitation applies to a comparison of SMR values. With full awareness of this limitation, it is interesting to note that using Table 5-1 data and the United States as the standard, $S\hat{M}R_b/S\hat{M}R_a$ = 1.125, $I\hat{S}R_b/I\hat{S}R_a$ = 1.125 (the ratio of two SMR values will always be identical to the ratio of the corresponding ISR values), and $D\hat{S}R_b/D\hat{S}R_a$ = 1.125. These are all in contrast to the corresponding ratio of crude rates, which is 1.337.

CONFOUNDING VARIABLES IN 2 × 2 TABLES

Tables 5-3 and 5-4 show data relating age, systolic blood pressure, and prevalence of myocardial infarction from a sample of the Israeli Ischemic Heart Disease Study population. We see that the odds ratios for disease comparing those with the factor and those without are 3.44 for age (Table 5-3) and 1.88 for blood pressure (Table 5-3). The odds ratio for higher blood pressure comparing older persons to younger is 3.04 (Table 5-4). If our major interest is in estimating the odds ratio relating systolic blood pressure to myocardial infarction, age is a confounding variable because it is related both to the disease of interest, myocardial infarction, and to the risk factor we wish to evaluate, systolic blood pressure. Thus the odds ratio of 1.88 relating elevated blood pressure to myocardial infarction risk reflects not only the association of blood pressure and myocardial infarction but also the association of age and myocardial infarction.

Stratification to Control Confounding

One obvious way to reduce the confounding effect of age is to look at the data in separate strata by age. Table 5-5 presents the data relating systolic blood pressure and myocardial infarction after they have been subdivided into age classes.

Interaction   The odds ratios in Table 5-5 relating elevated blood pressure to risk—0.95 for those age 60 and over and 1.87 for those under age 60—suggest a relationship between variables that we have not previously discussed. What meaning can be attached to an odds ratio relating high blood pressure to risk of disease if this odds ratio is different at different ages? Naturally the overall odds ratio can be viewed as an average derived from a combination of odds ratios for specific age classes. However, such an average would be interpreted one way if the items included were all sample estimates of the same odds ratio subject only

Table 5-3. Relationship of Age and Systolic Blood Pressure to Prevalence of Myocardial Infarction in a Sample of Individuals in the Israeli Ischemic Heart Disease Study

	Myocardial infarction	
	Present	Absent
Age ⩾ 60	15	188
Age < 60	41	1767 ($\hat{OR} = 3.44$)
SBP ⩾ 140	29	711
SBP < 140	27	1244 ($\hat{OR} = 1.88$)
Total	56	1955

Source: unpublished data from the Israeli Ischemic Heart Disease Study.

Table 5-4. Relationship of Systolic Blood Pressure to Age in a Sample of Individuals in the Israeli Ischemic Heart Disease Study

	Age $\geqslant 60$	Age < 60	Total
SBP $\geqslant 140$	124	616	740
SBP < 140	79	1192	1271
Total	203	1808	2011
			$\hat{OR} = 3.04$

Source: unpublished data from the Israeli Ischemic Heart Disease Study.

Table 5-5. Prevalence of Myocardial Infarction by Systolic Blood Pressure and Age

	MI cases	MI negative	Total
Age $\geqslant 60$			
SBP $\geqslant 140$	9 $(a_1)^a$	115 (b_1)	124 (m_{11})
SBP < 140	6 (c_1)	73 (d_1)	79 (m_{21})
Total	15 (n_{11})	188	203 (t_1)
			$\hat{OR} = 0.95$
Age < 60			
SBP $\geqslant 140$	20 (a_2)	596 (b_2)	616 (m_{12})
SBP < 140	21 (c_2)	1171 (d_2)	1192 (m_{22})
Total	41 (n_{12})	1767	1808 (t_2)
			$\hat{OR} = 1.87$

^{a}Letters in parentheses are used in the text discussion of these data.
Source: unpublished data from the Israeli Ischemic Heart Disease Study.

to random variation and another way if the odds ratios being averaged were truly different. If the association of blood pressure and risk is different at different ages (beyond the range of variation we can assign to chance), we say that there is *interaction* between age and blood pressure in relation to risk of disease. Miettinen suggests *effect modification* as a better description than interaction [42]. However, since *effect modification* implies a real effect requiring data beyond those of the associations we are discussing and since *interaction* is a quite common term in the statistical and epidemiologic literature, I shall continue using it.

Interaction can be defined more precisely. For simplicity, we shall do this with respect to mortality rates as related to attribute variables A and B. We define four mortality rates as follows:

AB mortality rate associated with variables A and B when both are present
aB mortality rate associated with variable B present but A is absent
Ab mortality rate associated with variable A present but B is absent
ab mortality rate associated with variables A and B when both are absent

Using the above notations, interaction between A and B can be defined as the existence of nonzero values of

$$(AB - aB) - (Ab - ab)$$

This difference of differences compares the arithmetic effect of A on mortality rate when B is present $(AB - aB)$ with the arithmetic effect of A on mortality rate when B is absent $(Ab - ab)$. If $AB - aB = Ab - ab$, we say there is *no interaction* between A and B. More exactly, if we do not detect a significant difference between sample estimates of $AB - aB$ and $Ab - ab$, we can say we have no evidence of interaction.

Interaction can be defined with respect to alternative scalings of data [43], for example, a logarithmic effect: $(\log AB - \log aB) - (\log Ab - \log ab)$. This is zero if $AB/aB = Ab/ab$. Absence of interaction on a logarithmic scale suggests that the ratio effect of A is unchanged whether B is present or not. Thus if A increases mortality rate by .10 whether or not B is present, then interaction between A and B is not present *when interaction is defined arithmetically*. However, if the increase of .10 is from .05 to .15 with B absent and from .20 to .30 with B present, AB interaction exists if it is defined on a logarithmic scale because the ratios .15/.05 and .30/.20 are unequal. Rothman has suggested a probability scale as biologically appropriate [44]. Additional discussion may be found in Schlesselman [45].

A final comment about interaction. If the effect of high blood pressure on mortality is considerable at younger ages and less so at older ages, that is a fact of nature we should try to uncover. It is not something we want to eliminate by clever transformation of the measurement scale [46]. Interaction between age and blood pressure is separate and distinct from confounding between age and blood pressure. If we do not properly control the latter, we overstate the effect of elevated blood pressure on mortality risk (because those with elevated pressure are older than those without it). To recapitulate the discussion of the relationship of age, blood pressure and risk:

1. Elimination of confounding between age and blood pressure with respect to risk results in better estimates of the overall association of blood pressure and risk.
2. If interaction between age and blood pressure is present, this estimate of the association between overall blood pressure and risk is not applicable to all age groups.

Mantel-Haenszel Procedure to Control Confounding

We now return to the data of Table 5-5 with estimated odds ratios for each of two age classes. The Mantel-Haenszel (M-H) procedure [47] can combine the odds ratios for separate strata into an overall summary estimate of the odds ratio relating blood pressure and risk of myocardial infarction. The advantage of this M-H overall odds ratio over the odds ratio for the same disease and risk factor given in Table 5-3, is that the confounding effect of age (with respect to two age classes) is eliminated. If there is a common odds ratio, the M-H procedure estimates it. If there is no common odds ratio (i.e., interaction is present), the M-H procedure provides a weighted average of the separate odds ratios. The overall odds ratio using the M-H procedure is estimated as follows:

$$\hat{OR} \text{ (overall)} = \frac{\sum_i a_i d_i / t_i}{\sum_i b_i c_i / t_i} \tag{5-17}$$

where t_i is the total number of individuals and $a_i d_i$ and $b_i c_i$ are the cross-product terms for the ith 2×2 table arranged as in Table 3-3. For the data in Table 5-5 this is

$$\frac{(9 \times 73)/203 + (20 \times 1171)/1808}{(115 \times 6)/203 + (596 \times 21)/1808} = 1.57$$

Thus, instead of estimating 1.88 as the odds ratio relating elevated systolic blood pressure to myocardial infarction prevalence, we now estimate it as 1.57 after removing part of the confounding effect of age. Presumably, the effect of age has not been eliminated entirely because *within* the age classes ≥ 60 and < 60 the persons with elevated blood pressure are likely to be older than the others. If this residual confounding is considered important, it can be dealt with by constructing additional age strata using narrower intervals or by multi-variate methods (described in Chapter 6).

Matching Data in 2 × 2 Tables

Another method for removing the confounding effects of age on the association of systolic blood pressure with myocardial infarction is to match each infarction case with one or more randomly chosen control *of the same age as the case.** Using unpublished data, we selected one control per case by picking an individual of the same age as the myocardial infarction case but without any history of myocardial infarction from a list of Israel Ischemic Heart Study participants arranged by age and serial number. The serial numbers were assigned in a way completely unrelated to age or blood pressure, and thus the qualifying individual with the next higher serial number than the case was a satisfactory choice. Data for the 56 *pairs* of matched cases and controls are summarized in Table 5-6. Note that Table 5-6 relates to pairs of individuals and not to single persons, i.e., 15 cases *and* 15 age-matched controls are represented by the 15 in the upper left corner of the table. Because Table 5-6 counts pairs and not individuals, the cells have different meaning than the cells in the 2 × 2 tables we have seen up to this point. For this reason the estimation of an odds ratio based on matched data is different from the usual calculation

Table 5-6. Relationship of Systolic Blood Pressure to Myocardial Infarction: Paired Case-Control Data Matched by Age

Cases	Controls		
	SBP $\geqslant 140$	SBP < 140	Total
SBP $\geqslant 140$	15	13	28
SBP < 140	11	17	28
Total	26	30	56

$$\hat{OR} = \frac{13}{11} = 1.18$$

Source: unpublished data from the Israeli Ischemic Heart Disease Study.

using the cross-products ratio. Before discussing the formula, it will be helpful to consider what information is provided about the relationship between systolic blood pressure and myocardial infarction by the 32 pairs in Table 5-6 (15 + 17), wherein the case and the control are in the *same* blood pressure category.

If you wish to study whether systolic blood pressure $\geqslant 140$ is positively associated with myocardial infarction, you cannot do so in a population in which everyone has systolic blood pressure $\geqslant 140$. The 32 pairs with case and control in the same blood pressure category similarly provide no basis for learning about how blood pressure might be related to myocardial infarction. If all individuals in a sample have high blood pressure or all have low blood pressure, it is impossible to learn from such a sample what might be the association between systolic blood pressure and myocardial infarction if blood pressure differences existed.

Another illustration may be useful. If you wish to discriminate between two swimmers as to which has a greater ability to swim long distances and you are given the following data on paired trials:

Trial 1   Both finished the prescribed course.
Trial 2   Both finished the prescribed course.
Trial 3   Neither finished the prescribed course.
Trial 4   A finished but B did not.

it should be clear that no judgment can be made as to greater endurance of one swimmer over the other from trials 1 through 3. Only trial 4, where there is a difference between the members of the pair, provides evidence as to possible difference between them. Similarly with the matched data. Pairs with both case and control having the risk factor or pairs with neither having the risk factor provide no information regarding the odds ratio. Data from a matched case-control study can be arranged as in Table 5-7, in which f is the number of *pairs* with both case and control factor positive, g is the number of *pairs* with the case factor positive and the control factor negative, etc. To emphasize that these are

Table 5-7. Case-Control Data for Matched Pairs

	Controls	
Cases	Risk factor +	Risk factor −
Risk factor + Risk factor −	f h	g j

paired data, we use the symbols f, g, h, j for cells of this 2×2 table to distinguish them from the a, b, c, d symbols we have used to represent unpaired data.

With data as in Table 5-7, the estimated odds ratio relating positive factor to presence of disease based on matched pairs (MP) is

$$\hat{OR} \text{ (MP)} = \frac{g}{h} \tag{5-18}$$

For the data in Table 5-6,

$$\frac{g}{h} = \frac{13}{11} = 1.18$$

As previously discussed, f and j contribute nothing to odds ratio estimation.

Recalling the M-H formula (Equation 5-17) for the overall odds ratio and applying it to matched pair data in which each pair is treated as a separate stratum also results in the ratio g/h as the estimated odds ratio for paired data. To see this, the paired data first have to be changed to their unpaired equivalent, as shown in Tables 5-8 through 5-11. The M-H formula for $\hat{OR}$,

$$\frac{\sum_i a_i d_i/t_i}{\sum_i b_i c_i/t_i}$$

applied to the data in Tables 5-8 to 5-11 will

Table 5-8. Conversion of Paired Data to Unpaired Equivalent When Both Case and Control Are Positive for Risk Factor

	Paired data		Unpaired equivalent		
	Controls				
Cases	Risk factor +	Risk factor −	Risk factor	Cases	Controls
Risk factor + Risk factor −	1 0	0 0	+ −	1 (a) 0 (c)	1 (b) 0 (d)
			$ad = 0, bc = 0, t = 2$		

1. Have zero added to the numerator and to the denominator for each pair with case and control alike ($a_i d_i = 0, b_i c_i = 0, t_i = 2$), as in Tables 5-8 and 5-11.
2. Have $\frac{1}{2}$ added to the numerator for each pair with the case positive and the control negative for the risk factor ($a_i d_i = 1, b_i c_i = 0, t_i = 2$), as in Table 5-9. There are g pairs of this type.

Table 5-9. Conversion of Paired Data to Unpaired Equivalent When Case Is Risk-Factor-Positive and Control Is Risk-Factor-Negative

	Paired data		Unpaired equivalent		
	Controls				
Cases	Risk factor +	Risk factor −	Risk factor	Cases	Controls
Risk factor +	0	1	+	1 (a)	0 (b)
Risk factor −	0	0	−	0 (c)	1 (d)
			$ad = 1, bc = 0, t = 2$		

Table 5-10. Conversion of Paired Data to Unpaired Equivalent When Case Is Risk-Factor-Negative and Control Is Risk-Factor-Positive

	Paired data		Unpaired equivalent		
	Controls				
Cases	Risk factor +	Risk factor −	Risk factor	Cases	Controls
Risk factor +	0	0	+	0 (a)	1 (b)
Risk factor −	1	0	−	1 (c)	0 (d)
			$ad = 0, bc = 1, t = 2$		

Table 5-11. Conversion of Paired Data to Unpaired Equivalent When Both Case and Control Are Negative for Risk Factor

	Paired data		Unpaired equivalent		
	Controls				
Cases	Risk factor +	Risk factor −	Risk factor	Cases	Controls
Risk factor +	0	0	+	0 (a)	0 (b)
Risk factor −	0	1	−	1 (c)	1 (d)
			$ad = 0, bc = 0, t = 2$		

3. Have $\frac{1}{2}$ added to the denominator for each pair with the case negative and the control positive for the risk factor ($a_i d_i = 0, b_i c_i = 1, t_i = 2$), as in Table 5-10. There are h pairs of this type.
4. Consequently equal $(g/2)/(h/2) = g/h$, as in Equation 5-18.

To recapitulate, we estimated the odds ratio for the association of myocardial infarction to elevated systolic blood pressure as 1.88 with no adjustment for confounding by age and as 1.57 after partially adjusting for age by stratifying the data into age $\geqslant$ 60 and age < 60. When we adjusted by means of individual matching on age, necessarily using only a subset of the full sample, the odds ratio was 1.18. Of course, sampling error is implicit in all these calculations, and it is possible that a method of adjustment that on average lowers an estimated odds ratio by reducing the effect of a confounding variable may in a specific instance actually raise it.

Before additional discussion of these estimated odds ratios for the relationship of myocardial infarction prevalence to elevated systolic blood pressure, it is first necessary to consider their relationship to odds ratios for myocardial infarction *incidence* in relation to elevated systolic blood pressure. Chapter 3 stressed that retrospective case-control studies are necessarily restricted to the use of prevalent cases. Because myocardial infarction is a disease with a high fatality rate, with sudden death as a not uncommon first manifestation, it should be obvious that the odds for *being* a case or *not being* a case based on existing cases may be quite different from the odds for *becoming* a case or *not becoming* a case based on prospective incidence data. In fact, incidence data from the same Israel Ischemic Heart Disease Study sample we have used here for prevalence associations do indicate larger odds ratios relating systolic blood pressure and incidence of myocardial infarction (adjusted for age) than those for prevalence. This may or may not be an important distinction for other diseases, and I include this comment to remind the reader to always consider the potential differences between data obtained prospectively and those obtained retrospectively.

CONFIDENCE LIMITS FOR ADJUSTED ODDS RATIOS

To discuss confidence limits for adjusted odds ratios, it is necessary to return to unmatched data in the (by now familiar) format of Table 3-3, except that we use a_i, b_i, c_i, and d_i to indicate sample data for the ith stratum. We shall use Woolf's method [20] to derive confidence limits on an overall estimate of the odds ratio and also to test whether or not interaction is present. For data sets as large as are usually available in high-quality epidemiologic studies, Woolf's method can be expected to give good results. However, other methods are available, including many programmed for a desk calculator [48]. For small data sets a statistician's advice will be helpful. In a later section we shall compare various alternative methods for calculating confidence limits on odds ratios, with particular attention to the size of the data set required for satisfactory results. If the reader will accept the estimated variance of $\ln \hat{OR}$ given by Woolf as

$$\frac{1}{a} + \frac{1}{b} + \frac{1}{c} + \frac{1}{d}$$

the remainder of his method for computing confidence intervals can be easily derived.

Logarithms are used to calculate confidence limits on odds ratios because they introduce approximate normality into the otherwise extremely skewed distribution of all possible sample odds ratios. Thus while an $\hat{OR}$ of 3 is farther from its expected value of unity (under the null hypothesis) than is an $\hat{OR}$ of $1/3$, $\ln 3$ $(= 1.0986)$ is exactly as far from its expected value of zero (under the null hypothesis) as is $\ln (1/3)$ $(= -1.0986)$. In combining $\ln \hat{OR}_i$ values for individual strata into a single overall estimate, it is sensible to give more weight to those $\ln \hat{OR}_i$ that are estimated with greater precision. An easy way to accomplish this is to weight each $\ln \hat{OR}_i$ by

$$\left(\frac{1}{a_i} + \frac{1}{b_i} + \frac{1}{c_i} + \frac{1}{d_i} \right)^{-1}$$

the reciprocal of its estimated variance. If we designate this reciprocal as w_i, we have

$$\ln \hat{OR} = \frac{\sum\limits_i w_i \ln \hat{OR}_i}{\sum\limits_i w_i} \tag{5-19}$$

Making use of Equations 1-8 and 1-10, the variance of $\ln OR$ is

$$\hat{var}(\ln OR) = \frac{\sum\limits_i w_i^2 [\hat{var}(\ln OR_i)]}{\left(\sum\limits_i w_i \right)^2}$$

But since

$$w_i = \frac{1}{\hat{var}(\ln OR_i)} \qquad \hat{var}(\ln OR_i) = \frac{1}{w_i}$$

and

$$\hat{var}(\ln OR) = \frac{\sum\limits_i w_i^2 \left(\frac{1}{w_i} \right)}{\left(\sum\limits_i w_i \right)^2} = \frac{\sum\limits_i w_i}{\left(\sum\limits_i w_i \right)^2} = \frac{1}{\sum\limits_i w_i} \tag{5-20}$$

the estimated standard error of $\ln \hat{OR}$ is then $1/\sqrt{\sum w_i}$, and 95 percent confidence limits on $\ln OR$ are

$$\ln \hat{OR} \pm 1.96\left(\frac{1}{\sqrt{\sum\limits_i w_i}}\right) \tag{5-21}$$

After finding the 95 percent confidence limits on $\ln OR$, the corresponding antilogs,

$$e^{\ln \hat{OR} \,-\, (1.96/\sqrt{\sum w_i})} \qquad e^{\ln \hat{OR} \,+\, (1.96/\sqrt{\sum w_i})} \tag{5-22}$$

are the 95 percent confidence limits on OR.

If we are thinking about combining odds ratios from separate strata, it is useful to test for interaction. Consider the data in Table 5-5. The odds ratios for the two strata are .95 and 1.87. Perhaps the odds ratio of .95 reflects a true odds ratio of 1.00 for age < 60 and the odds ratio of 1.87 reflects a true odds ratio of 2.00 for age $\geqslant 60$. If the underlying odds ratios for individual strata are really different, do we want to calculate an overall average value? In any event, we should determine whether or not the strata odds ratios reflect basic differences. A test for interaction on Table 5-5 data (i.e., is the effect of blood pressure on risk different at different ages?) will answer the question as to whether it is desirable to combine individual odds ratios.

A systematic summary of Table 5-5 data, which we shall use to test for interaction and also to compute confidence limits, can be prepared as shown in Table 5-12. Using these summary data from Table 5-12, we have

$$\ln \hat{OR} = \frac{3.33(-.0513) + 10.00(.6259)}{3.33 + 10.00} = .4567$$

$$\hat{OR} = e^{.4567} = 1.58$$

To test for interaction, we use Equation 1-22 for χ^2_{k-1}. This helps us to determine if the individual $\ln \hat{OR}_i$ for each stratum differs from $\ln \hat{OR}$ by more than can be explained by random variation. For this specific problem, χ^2 is

Table 5-12. Systematic Summary of Functions of Data Taken From Table 5-5

Stratum	$\hat{OR}_i$	$\ln \hat{OR}_i$	vâr $(\ln OR_i)$	$1/$vâr $(\ln OR_i) = w_i$
1	.95	$-.0513$	$\dfrac{1}{9} + \dfrac{1}{6} + \dfrac{1}{115} + \dfrac{1}{73} = .300$	3.33
2	1.87	.6259	$\dfrac{1}{20} + \dfrac{1}{21} + \dfrac{1}{596} + \dfrac{1}{1171} = .100$	10.00

computed as follows:

$$\chi^2_{2-1} = \sum_{i=1}^{2} \frac{(\ln \hat{OR}_i - \ln \hat{OR})^2}{\text{var}(\ln \hat{OR}_i)}$$

Our test for interaction on the two odds ratios shown in Table 5-5 data is then

$$\chi^2_1 = \frac{(-.0513 - .4567)^2}{.300} + \frac{(.6259 - .4567)^2}{.100} = 1.15$$

Since the probability of a χ^2_1 value of 1.15 or greater is more than 20 percent, we lack evidence that the odds ratios in Table 5-5, different as they are (.95 and 1.87), are not sample values from the same population. Thus the overall odds ratio of 1.58 may be interpreted as indicating the general relationship between systolic blood pressure elevation and risk of myocardial infarction.

Of course, it should be recognized that with only 15 cases of myocardial infarction in the age ≥ 60 group, the ability of our interaction test to detect, in the odds ratios in different strata, a difference greater than can be accounted for by chance is quite modest. The technical term for the ability of sample data to detect differences if they exist is *power*. Obviously, other factors being equal, the smaller the sample, the less power $(1 - \beta)$ to detect differences if they are present.

Since we lack evidence of interaction, it is certainly reasonable to make use of the overall estimates of OR previously calculated. We illustrate the calculation of confidence limits for $\ln \hat{OR}$ using Equation 5-21 and Table 5-5 data as summarized in Table 5-12:

$$\ln \hat{OR} = .4567$$

$$\hat{SE}(\ln OR) = \frac{1}{(\sum w_i)^{1/2}} = \frac{1}{(3.33 + 10.00)^{1/2}} = .2739$$

95% CL on $\ln OR = .4567 \pm 1.96(.2739) = -.0801$ and $.9935$

95% CL on $OR = e^{-.0801}$ and $e^{.9935} = .92$ and 2.70

We now discuss an alternative to Woolf's method for calculating confidence limits on an overall odds ratio derived from a combination of odds ratios for separate strata. This procedure, which is based on a significance test, was suggested by Miettinen [49], and we shall use it in combination with the M-H procedure [47] for estimating an overall odds ratio and testing it for significance.

First consider the M-H χ^2 test (one degree of freedom) on the data in a set of 2×2 tables. The χ^2_1 indicates whether or not the data are unusual in terms of deviation from expectation under the null hypothesis, which is that disease and risk factor are related only by chance. Any other χ_1^2 test of the *same data* with respect to the *same null hypothesis* should indicate the same degree of unusualness, i.e., the same χ_1^2 value. If the sample size is adequate, any test of departure from the null hypothesis should lead to the same χ_1^2 value because with only one degree of freedom it is not possible to measure departure from expectation in more than one basic way. Thus whether, as in the M-H χ_1^2 test, relating $\sum a_i$ to $\mathrm{E}(\sum a_i)$ and dividing by $\mathrm{var}(\sum a_i)$ or, as I now propose, relating $\ln \hat{OR}$ to $\mathrm{E}(\ln \hat{OR})$ and dividing by $\mathrm{var}(\ln \hat{OR})$, χ_1^2 based on the same data should be equivalent. We are now ready to describe in detail and calculate the M-H χ_1^2 for Table 5-5 data.

The overall significance test for a set of 2×2 tables suggested by Mantel and Haenszel [47] is

$$\chi_1^2 = \frac{[|\sum a_i - \mathrm{E}(\sum a_i)| - \frac{1}{2}]^2}{\mathrm{var}(\sum a_i)} \tag{5-23}$$

This formula is basically the same as Equation 1-21 with

$$x = \sum a_i$$

$$\mathrm{E}(x) = \mathrm{E}(\sum a_i) = \sum (\mathrm{E}a_i)$$

$$\mathrm{var}(x) = \mathrm{var}(\sum a_i) = \sum [\mathrm{var}(a_i)]$$

Note that because the a_i in separate strata are independent, the variance of the sum of the a_i values equals the sum of the variances of the a_i values. In addition, the expected value of a sum is always the sum of the expected values, whether or not the variables are independent. If we use the notation of Table 3-3 we have

$$x = \sum a_i$$

$$\mathrm{E}(x) = \mathrm{E}(\sum a_i) = \sum (\mathrm{E}a_i) = \sum \left(n_{1i}\frac{m_{1i}}{t_i}\right)$$

i.e., under the null hypothesis, the expected number of cases in stratum i with risk factor present equals the total number of cases (n_{1i}) multiplied by the proportion with the risk factor among cases and noncases combined (m_{1i}/t_i). Under the assumption that row and column totals in each stratum are fixed and not subject to sampling error, the variance of a_i is

$$n_{1i}\left(\frac{m_{1i}}{t_i}\right)\left(\frac{m_{2i}}{t_i}\right)\left(\frac{t_i - n_{1i}}{t_{i-1}}\right)$$

The above is analogous to the variance of a binomial sum, given in Equation 1-18, but with the finite correction factor added; thus

$$np(1 - p)\left(\frac{N - n}{N - 1}\right)$$

For the data at hand

$$n = n_{1i}$$

$$p = m_{1i}/t_i$$

$$(1 - p) = m_{2i}/t_i$$

$$N = t_i$$

then

$$\sum \text{var}(a_i) = \sum n_{1i}\left(\frac{m_{1i}}{t_i}\right)\left(\frac{m_{2i}}{t_i}\right)\left(\frac{t_i - n_{1i}}{t_i - 1}\right)$$

The final element in Equation 5-23 is the reduction of the absolute value of the difference between $\sum a_i$ observed and $\sum a_i$ expected by one half before squaring. This represents the continuity correction for χ^2 intended to make the integral values in a 2×2 table fit more closely to the continuous variable represented by the χ^2 distribution. This continuity correction is due to Yates [50].

To compute the M-H summary odds ratio and χ_1^2 test pertaining to it, we use the data of Table 5-5 according to the labeling shown therein. Then, as previously calculated,

$$\hat{OR}_{\text{M-H}} = \frac{\sum a_i d_i / t_i}{\sum b_i c_i / t_i} = \frac{9(73)/203 + 20(1171)/1808}{115(6)/203 + 596(21)/1808} = 1.57$$

and for the M-H χ_1^2

$$x = \sum a_i = 9 + 20 = 29$$

$$E(x) = \sum(Ea_i) = \frac{15(124)}{203} + \frac{41(616)}{1808} = 23.13$$

$$\text{var} x = \text{var}\left(\sum a_i\right) = \sum(\text{var} a_i) = 15\left(\frac{124}{203}\right)\left(\frac{79}{203}\right)\left(\frac{203 - 15}{203 - 1}\right)$$

$$+ 41\left(\frac{616}{1808}\right)\left(\frac{1192}{1808}\right)\left(\frac{1808 - 41}{1808 - 1}\right) = 12.32$$

$$\chi_1^2 = \frac{[|29 - 23.13| - \frac{1}{2}]^2}{12.32} = 2.34$$

We now use the value of $\chi_1^2 = 2.34$ as equal to another χ_1^2, one that, at least conceptually, could have been calculated from these data, namely

$$\chi_1^2 = \frac{[\ln \hat{OR}_{M\text{-}H} - E(\ln \hat{OR}_{M\text{-}H})]^2}{\text{var}(\ln \hat{OR}_{M\text{-}H})} = 2.34$$

Because we do not know the formula for var $(\ln \hat{OR}_{M\text{-}H})$, we cannot calculate the above directly. However, the use of χ_1^2 from another significance test on these data allows us to proceed as follows. Since the $\hat{OR}_{M\text{-}H}$ was 1.57, $\ln \hat{OR}$ can be calculated as $\ln 1.57 = .4511$. Under the null hypothesis, the expected value of $OR_{M\text{-}H} = 1$ and thus the expected value of $\ln \hat{OR}_{M\text{-}H}$ is zero and we have

$$\chi_1^2 = \frac{(.4511 - 0)^2}{\text{var}(\ln \hat{OR}_{M\text{-}H})} = 2.34$$

This equation can then be solved for var $(\ln \hat{OR}_{M\text{-}H})$, which is found to equal .0870. Note that this value for var $(\ln \hat{OR}_{M\text{-}H})$ has been derived not directly from any considerations as to the sampling distribution of $\ln \hat{OR}_{M\text{-}H}$ but from the equivalence of two possible expressions for χ_1^2 based on departure of Table 5-5 data from the null hypothesis. Because of the manner in which we obtained it, this variance of $\ln \hat{OR}_{M\text{-}H}$ is strictly applicable only under null hypothesis conditions, i.e., $OR_{M\text{-}H} = 1$ and $\ln OR_{M\text{-}H} = 0$ [51]. As a practical matter, it has been found useful over a fairly wide range of departures from the null hypothesis, and you need not hesitate to use it.

With var$(\ln \hat{OR}_{M\text{-}H})$ as .0870, the standard error of $\ln \hat{OR}_{M\text{-}H}$ is $(.0870)^{1/2}$ = .2950 and 95 percent confidence limits on $\ln OR_{M\text{-}H}$ can be estimated as

$$\ln \hat{OR}_{M\text{-}H} \pm 1.96(.2950) = .4511 \pm .5782$$

$$95\% \text{ CL on } \ln OR_{M\text{-}H} \doteq -.1271 \text{ and } 1.0293$$

$$95\% \text{ CL on } OR_{M\text{-}H} = e^{-.1271} \text{ and } e^{1.0293} = .88 \text{ and } 2.80$$

Note the close agreement between Miettinen's method and Woolf's method for estimating a common odds ratio and its confidence limits. For the common odds ratio Woolf's method estimated 1.58 and the M-H procedure estimated 1.57. The 95 percent confidence limits derived from Woolf's method were .92 and 2.70, versus .88 and 2.80 from Miettinen's test-based procedure using the M-H summary odds ratio and χ_1^2 test for significance. A point to emphasize is that the essential equivalence of the two approaches in this particular instance relates to 2 × 2 tables with cells as small as 6 and 9. If the basic data were more substantial, we would expect even closer agreement. As an indication of this, if all cell frequencies in Table 5-5 were doubled, the confidence limits on OR using Woolf's method would be 1.08 and 2.31, barely distinguishable from the 1.06 and 2.32 obtained from the test-based procedure of Miettinen.

Although a recent analysis [52] concludes that the Cornfield method referred to in Chapter 3 is superior to both Woolf's method and Miettinen's test-based method for estimating confidence limits on odds ratios derived from single 2 × 2 tables, the data shown in that report agree completely with my own experience that differences are not important. The only large difference reported among the three methods is for the interval .18 and 5.49 versus .26 and 9.45. Clearly either of these confidence limits makes the same point, i.e., that we are almost completely ignorant about the size of the true odds ratio.

We now consider another example illustrating the use of the test-based procedure for confidence limits. For matched pair data arranged as in Table 5-7 and using $\hat{OR}$ (MP) to represent the estimated odds ratio from matched pair data, the proper estimate of OR (MP) is g/h, as in Equation 5-18.

The M-H χ^2 test to evaluate whether OR (MP) is significantly different from unity depends on whether g is significantly different from $\frac{1}{2}(g + h)$. Under the condition that the test relates only to samples in which the total number of discordant pairs equals $g + h$, the number of discordant pairs actually observed, the M-H χ_1^2 is exactly equivalent to Equation 1-21 as applied to a binomial variable and uses

g as the number of successes observed in $g + h$ trials
$\frac{1}{2}(g + h)$ as the expected number of successes
$g + h$ as the number of trials
$(g + h)(\frac{1}{2})(\frac{1}{2})$ as the variance of the number of successes observed

Then

$$\chi_1^2 = \frac{\left(g - \dfrac{g + h}{2}\right)^2}{(g + h)(\frac{1}{2})(\frac{1}{2})} = \frac{\left(\dfrac{g}{2} - \dfrac{h}{2}\right)^2 4}{g + h} = \frac{(g - h)^2}{g + h}$$

and using the continuity correction, the M-H χ_1^2 for testing if $\hat{OR}$ (MP) is significantly different from unity is

$$\chi_1^2 = \frac{(|g - h| - 1)^2}{g + h} \tag{5-24}$$

For Table 5-6 data, this is

$$\chi_1^2 = \frac{(|13 - 11| - 1)^2}{13 + 11} = \frac{1}{24} = .042$$

clearly not a large departure from expectation under the null hypothesis.

Recalling that $\hat{OR}$ (MP) from Table 5-6 is 1.18, we can now use Equation 1-

21 with $\ln \hat{OR}$ (MP) substituted for x and solve for SE $[\ln \hat{OR}$ (MP)]:

$$\chi_1^2 = \frac{(\ln \hat{OR} \text{ (MP)} - 0)^2}{\text{var}[\ln \hat{OR} \text{ (MP)}]} = \frac{(.1655 - 0)^2}{\text{var}[\ln \hat{OR} \text{ (MP)}]} = .042$$

$$\text{var}[\ln \hat{OR} \text{ (MP)}] = .6521$$

$$\text{SE}[\ln \hat{OR} \text{ (MP)}] = .8076$$

and the 95 percent confidence limits on $\ln OR$ (MP) are

$$\ln \hat{OR} \text{ (MP)} \pm 1.96(.8076) = .1655 \pm 1.5829 = -1.4174 \text{ and } 1.7484$$

The corresponding antilogs, $e^{-1.4174}$ and $e^{1.7484}$, are .24 and 5.75. These are the 95 percent confidence limits on the OR (MP) derived from Table 5-6.

This general procedure for test-based confidence limits can be applied in many other instances as well. Of course, original values rather than logarithms would be used if the statistic used in the calculation of confidence limits for a given parameter was itself approximately normally distributed.

MULTIPLE MATCHED CONTROLS

Matching K controls to each case, where K may be 2, 3, or possibly even larger, is sometimes done when controls are available at much lower cost than cases. This procedure is also sometimes used in an effort to obtain the maximum information possible from a case-control comparison when only a small number of cases are available. If we cross-classify each set consisting of a case and its K matched controls, as in Table 5-13, we can consider each set as a separate stratum and calculate the odds ratio using Equation 5-17.

In Table 5-13 we use the a_i, b_i, c_i, d_i, t_i designations previously described. However, we have used total row and column symbols appropriate to matching K controls per case. Thus, $a_i + c_i = 1$, $b_i + d_i = K$, and $t_i = 1 + K$. We again use the M-H procedure to combine sets and to estimate the overall odds ratio as $\dfrac{\sum (a_i d_i)/t_i}{\sum (b_i c_i)/t_i}$. Comparable to the case of one-to-one matching, zero will be added to $\sum (a_i d_i)/t_i$ and to $\sum (b_i c_i)/t_i$ if the case and all controls are all factor-

Table 5-13. Notation for Matched Case and K Controls (i th Set)

	Case	Controls	Total
Risk factor +	a_i	b_i	$a_i + b_i$
Risk factor −	c_i	d_i	$1 + K - a_i - b_i$
Total	1	K	$1 + K$ (t_i)

Table 5-14. Data Summary in 2×2 Table for Each Set of Two Controls and One Case with Case Positive and Both Controls Negative[a,b]

	MI case	Control	Total
SBP $\geqslant$ 140	1	0	1
SBP $<$ 140	0	2	2
Total	1	2	3

$K = 2, ad = 2, bc = 0, Ka - b = 2, (a + b)(1 + K - a - b) = 2, ad/t = 2/3$

[a] Eleven sets of this type; see text.
[b] See Table 5-13 for explanation of notation.
Source: unpublished data from the Israeli Ischemic Heart Disease Study.

Table 5-15. Data Summary in 2×2 Table for Each Set of Two Controls and One Case with Case Positive and One Control Positive, One Negative[a,b]

	MI case	Control	Total
SBP $\geqslant$ 140	1	1	2
SBP $<$ 140	0	1	1
Total	1	2	3

$K = 2, ad = 1, bc = 0, Ka - b = 1, (a + b)(1 + K - a - b) = 2, ad/t = 1/3$

[a] Nine sets of this type; see text.
[b] See Table 5-13 for explanation of notation.
Source: unpublished data from the Israeli Ischemic Heart Disease Study.

positive or all factor-negative. Either $a_i d_i/t_i$ or $b_i c_i/t_i$ will have nonzero values whenever case and controls show disagreement as to proportion with the factor positive, e.g., case is factor positive and at least one control is factor negative.

Returning to the 56 myocardial infarction cases from our sample from the Israeli Ischemic Heart Disease Study population, we randomly matched each case with two controls and calculated the odds ratio. The data consist of 11 triplets as in Table 5-14, 9 triplets as in Table 5-15, 11 triplets as in Table 5-16, and 5 triplets as in Table 5-17. Eight triplets were all factor-positive, and 12 were all factor-negative. These 20 triplets provided no information as to the odds ratio and are excluded from the calculations. In Tables 5-14 to 5-17 are also shown some derivative values needed for the significance test to be described.

The odds ratio based on data from Tables 5-14 through 5-17 computed using Equation 5-17 is

$$\hat{OR}\ (MK) = \frac{11(2/3) + 9(1/3)}{11(1/3) + 5(2/3)} = \frac{31}{21} = 1.48$$

Table 5-16. Data Summary in 2×2 Table for Each Set of Two Controls and One Case with Case Negative and One Control Positive, One Negative[a, b]

	MI case	Control	Total
SBP $\geqslant$ 140	0	1	1
SBP < 140	1	1	2
Total	1	2	3

$K = 2$, $ad = 0$, $bc = 1$, $Ka - b = -1$, $(a + b)(1 + K - a - b) = 2$, $bc/t = 1/3$

[a] Eleven sets of this type; see text.
[b] See Table 5-13 for explanation of notation.
Source: unpublished data from the Israeli Ischemic Heart Disease Study.

Table 5-17. Data Summary in 2×2 Table for Each Set of Two Controls and One Case with Case Negative and Both Controls Positive[a, b]

	MI case	Control	Total
SBP $\geqslant$ 140	0	2	2
SBP < 140	1	0	1
Total	1	2	3

$K = 2$, $ad = 0$, $bc = 2$, $Ka - b = -2$, $(a + b)(1 + K - a - b) = 2$, $bc/t = 2/3$

[a] Five sets of this type; see text.
[b] See Table 5-13 for explanation of notation.
Source: unpublished data from the Israeli Ischemic Heart Disease Study.

with $\hat{OR}\,(MK)$ used to indicate an estimated odds ratio based on matching K controls per case. A significance test comparing cases and controls that are factor-positive, in matched data with K controls for each case, is given by Miettinen [53] as

$$z = \sum_i (Ka_i - b_i) \Big/ \left[\sum_i (a_i + b_i)(1 + K - a_i - b_i) \right]^{1/2} \qquad (5\text{-}25)$$

where z is a standardized normal deviate if the null hypothesis, that $\hat{OR}\,(MK) = 1$, is true.

Although different in appearance, Equation 5-25 is derived in a manner similar to that used to derive the M-H summary χ_1^2. We begin by establishing the statistic for testing departure from expectation if there is no difference between cases and controls in the proportion positive for the risk factor under study. As with the M-H χ_1^2, we shall focus upon the number of cases positive for the risk factor in each set (stratum), i.e., a_i in Table 5-13. In this matched design, a_i is either 1 or 0. Under the null hypothesis, a_i is *not* expected to equal b_i, which is the number of controls positive for the risk factor, because our design calls for K controls per case. Thus, with no relationship between disease and risk factor, we do not expect a_i to be as large as b_i. On the average, however, we would expect Ka_i to be as large as b_i. Our test statistic is then $Ka_i - b_i$, which has an expected value of zero under the null hypothesis. The next step is to derive the standard error of the test statistic, and we do so under the condition that, in each set, row and column totals are fixed and not subject to sampling variation. The statistic to be tested for significance contains two variables, a_i and b_i, and because their total is a constant, it is easy enough to convert this to a form with just one variable:

$$Ka_i - b_i = Ka_i + (a_i + b_i) - b_i - (a_i + b_i) = (K + 1)a_i - (a_i + b_i)$$

Since $a_i + b_i$ is a constant, its sampling variance is zero and

$$\mathrm{var}(Ka_i - b_i) = \mathrm{var}[(K + 1)a_i] = (K + 1)^2 \, \mathrm{var}(a_i)$$

If we consider a_i in Table 5-13 as a binomial sum with estimated variance of $np(1 - p)$, as in Equation 1-18, or as $np(1 - p)(N - n)/(N - 1)$ if we include the finite sampling factor, then the equivalent notation from Table 5-13 is

$$n = 1 \quad p = \frac{a_i + b_i}{1 + K} \quad 1 - p = \frac{1 + K - a_i - b_i}{1 + K} \quad N = 1 + K$$

$$\mathrm{v\hat{a}r}(Ka_i - b_i) = (K + 1)^2 \left[1\left(\frac{a_i + b_i}{1 + K}\right) \frac{(1 + K - a_i - b_i)}{1 + K} \right]\left(\frac{1 + K - 1}{1 + K - 1}\right)$$

$$= (a_i + b_i)(1 + K - a_i - b_i)$$

Since the sets are independent, the estimated variance of $\sum (Ka_i - b_i)$ is $\sum (a_i + b_i)(1 + K - a_i - b_i)$ and dividing $\sum (Ka_i - b_i)$ by the square root of its variance leads to Equation 5-25 for a standardized normal deviate, as given by Miettinen [53].

Using data from Tables 5-14 through 5-17† and Equation 5-25,

$$z = \frac{11(2) + 9(1) + 11(-1) + 5(-2)}{[11(2) + 9(2) + 11(2) + 5(2)]^{1/2}} = \frac{10}{8.49} = 1.18$$

Since z is a standardized normal deviate, we use z^2 as equivalent to χ_1^2 in Miettinen's method for estimating a variance that might be difficult to estimate directly. Thus, under the null hypothesis

$$\frac{[\ln \hat{OR}(MK) - 0]^2}{\mathrm{var}[\ln \hat{OR}(MK)]} = z^2 = \chi_1^2$$

We have inserted zero for the expectation of $\ln \hat{OR}$ (MK) in this equation because, if OR (MK) = 1, then $\ln OR$ (MK) = 0. Inserting the values calculated for $\hat{OR}$ (MK) and z^2 for the Israeli sample data relating hypertension to myocardial infarction prevalence results in

$$\frac{(.3920 - 0)^2}{\mathrm{var}[\ln \hat{OR}\,(MK)]} = (1.18)^2 = 1.39$$

$$\mathrm{var}[\ln \hat{OR}(MK)] = .1105$$

$$\mathrm{SE}[\ln \hat{OR}\,(MK)] = .3324$$

and 95 percent confidence limits for $\ln OR$ (MK) are

$$(.3920) \pm 1.96(.3324) = .3920 \pm .6515 = -.2595 \text{ and } 1.0435$$

with $e^{-.2595}$ and $e^{1.0435}$, or .77 and 2.84, as the 95 percent confidence limits for OR (MK). As expected, these limits are narrower than the limits based on one control per case, which we earlier found to be .24 and 5.75.

In considering the value of multiple controls per case, it is useful to keep in mind that the essential component of a case-control study is the comparison of cases to controls with respect to the proportion having the risk factor. How effective multiple controls are in increasing the precision of this comparison is suggested by the following discussion.

Under the null hypothesis the proportion of cases with the risk factor equals the proportion of controls with the risk factor. If this proportion is P_0, the variance of the difference between cases and controls is

$$\frac{P_0 Q_0}{n_{\mathrm{cases}}} + \frac{P_0 Q_0}{n_{\mathrm{controls}}}$$

Suppose that the sample size for controls is K times as large as that for cases, so that

$$\mathrm{var}\,(p_{\mathrm{cases}} - p_{\mathrm{controls}}) = \frac{P_0 Q_0}{n} + \frac{P_0 Q_0}{Kn} = \frac{(K+1)}{K}\left(\frac{P_0 Q_0}{n}\right)$$

and $\quad \mathrm{SE}\,(p_{\mathrm{cases}} - p_{\mathrm{controls}}) = \left[\frac{K+1}{K}\left(\frac{P_0 Q_0}{n}\right)\right]^{1/2}$

If we use the standard error of the difference in p between cases and controls as a basis for comparison and compute the ratio

$$\frac{\text{SE based on } K \text{ controls per case}}{\text{SE based on one control per case}}$$

Table 5-18. Ratio of Standard Error of Difference Between p_{case} and $p_{control}$, Comparing n Cases and nk Controls with n Cases and n Controls

Controls per case (k)	$\dfrac{SE(p_{n\,cases} - p_{nk\,controls})}{SE(p_{n\,cases} - p_{n\,controls})}$
1	1.00
2	.87
3	.82
4	.79
5	.77

We can see how much the standard error is decreased with increasing number of controls ($2n$, $3n$, etc.). This is shown in Table 5-18. It is obvious that there is little gain in precision, i.e., reduction of $SE(p_{cases} - p_{controls})$, after $K = 2$. Values of K larger than 2 are probably not warranted unless control data are available at essentially no cost.

NOTES

* Matching can also be accomplished by considering age within $\pm\ x$ years, where the value of x depends upon the judgment of the investigator, i.e., matching within an age group.
† Those sets with the case and both controls alike as to presence of the risk factor contribute nothing to the value of z. They simply add zero to both numerator and denominator. The constant value of $(a_i + b_i)(1 + K - a_i - b_i) = 2$ for all relevant case-control sets is a peculiarity of Equation 5-25 for $K = 2$.

6

Adjustment Using Multiple Linear Regression and Multiple Logistic Functions

REVIEW OF SIMPLE LINEAR REGRESSION

The notation throughout this chapter refers to sample data and sample statistics unless specifically stated otherwise.

The simple linear regression equation

$$\hat{y} = a + bx \tag{6-1}$$

describes a linear relationship between x and y in which, for each unit increase in x, the estimated value of y increases on the average by b units and in which $\hat{y} = a$ when $x = 0$. For relevance to epidemiologic investigation, we shall assume that values of x and y are derived from a sample of individuals.

The specific numeric values of a and b are derived from the data by the method of least squares. The least-squares a and b values are those for which $\sum (y_j - \hat{y}_j)^2$ is a minimum, where $\hat{y}_j$ is the computed value of $a + bx_j$ for the jth individual and y_j is the actual value of y for the jth individual. Discussion of simple and multiple linear regression as well as formulas for regression coefficients and their standard error is available in most statistics texts [1,5].

MULTIPLE LINEAR REGRESSION COEFFICIENTS

Because b relates to the association of change in y with change in x, epidemiologists are usually more interested in b than in a, and we now investigate the meaning of b_1 and b_2 in a multiple regression equation in which coefficients have been determined by the method of least squares:

$$\hat{y} = a + b_1 x_1 + b_2 x_2 \tag{6-2}$$

It is often stated that b_1 reflects the relationship between x_1 and y when x_2 is "held constant." I have always felt this to be somewhat lacking in clarity, and I hope the following explanation will be an improvement. To clearly distinguish that a and b in the simple regression equations below are not necessarily the same as the a, b_1, and b_2 in Equation 6-2, I shall use $a'b'$, $a''b''$, etc., to distinguish them.

We can calculate simple linear least-squares regression coefficients between y and x_2 and then estimate y as follows:

$$\hat{y} = a' + b'x_2 \tag{6-3}$$

We can similarly calculate simple linear least-squares regression coefficients between x_1 and x_2 and then estimate x_1 as follows:

$$\hat{x}_1 = a'' + b''x_2 \tag{6-4}$$

Using Equation 6-3, we can then calculate, for each individual, the discrepancy between the observed value of y and the value of $\hat{y}$ computed on the basis of the linear relationship with x_2. Using Equation 6-4, we can also calculate, for each individual, the discrepancy between the observed value of x_1 and the value of $\hat{x}_1$ computed on the basis of the linear relationship with x_2. For the j th individual, these two discrepancies are

$$y_j - \hat{y}_{j(x_2)}$$
$$x_{1j} - \hat{x}_{1j(x_2)}$$

where $\hat{y}_{j(x_2)}$ represents an estimated value for y_j derived from the linear regression of y on x_2 and $\hat{x}_{1j(x_2)}$ represents an estimated value for x_{1j} derived from the linear regression of x_1 on x_2. Now, if we compute simple linear regression coefficients between the portion of y *not* linearly related to x_2 and the portion of x_1 *not* linearly related to x_2, i.e., between

$$y - \hat{y}_{(x_2)} \qquad \text{and} \qquad x_1 - \hat{x}_{1(x_2)},$$

we obtain least-squares simple regression coefficients a''' and b''' for the equation:

$$y - \hat{y}_{(x_2)} = a''' + b'''[x_1 - \hat{x}_{1(x_2)}] \tag{6-5}$$

Understanding of the meaning of coefficients in multiple regression equations is improved by realizing that b''' in Equation 6-5 is *exactly* equal to b_1 in Equation 6-2. The point to be emphasized is that in an equation such as

$$\hat{y} = a + b_1x_1 + b_2x_2 + b_3x_3 \tag{6-6}$$

b_1 indicates the average increase in y for a unit change in x_1 *after* the linear association with x_2 and x_3 has been removed from *both* x_1 and y. Similarly, b_2 indicates the average increase in y for a unit change in x_2 *after* linear association with x_1 and x_3 has been removed from *both* x_2 and y, etc. Thus, this method can be used to adjust for several confounding factors simultaneously. More generally, in multiple linear regression equations, the regression coefficient for x_i indicates an average change in y for a unit change in x_i after their linear association with all other x variables has been removed from both y and x_i.

Note that Equation 6-6 implies the absence of interaction among the x variables. If in fact interaction is important—if, for example, the change in y for a unit change in x_1 is quite different depending on whether x_2 is large or small—the agreement, or fit, of Equation 6-6 with the data is necessarily adversely affected. Under these conditions, the fit of the model (equation) to the data could be improved by adding a cross-product term, $b_4 x_1 x_2$, to Equation 6-6.

Table 6-1 presents data for the systolic blood pressures, ages, and weights of 15 individuals taken from a large epidemiologic study. These will be used to illustrate the relationship between simple and multiple linear regression.

Table 6-2 presents, for each of the 15 individuals listed in Table 6-1, (a) estimates of weight based on a simple linear regression with age, (b) estimates of systolic blood pressure based on a simple linear regression with age, and (c) estimates of systolic blood pressure based on multiple linear regression with age and weight. Alongside each of the estimated values in Table 6-2 is the discrepancy between the estimate and the actual value.

If we now calculate the simple regression between weight after removal of a component linearly related to age (column 2 in Table 6-2) as the independent

Table 6-1. Data Fragment from a Large Epidemiologic Study

Individual	Systolic blood pressure (mmHg)	Age (years)	Weight (lb)
1	132	49	145
2	155	56	216
3	130	52	115
4	142	46	170
5	150	57	172
6	128	42	166
7	126	43	164
8	118	45	152
9	180	56	275
10	124	52	221
11	150	42	175
12	134	57	132
13	140	56	188
14	142	56	178
15	128	53	168
Total	2079	762	2637

Table 6-2. Simple and Multiple Linear Regression Computations Derived from Table 6-1.

Individual	Weight = 80.859 + 1.869(age) (simple regression)		SBP = 81.900 + 1.116(age) (simple regression)		SBP = 61.844 + 0.653(age) + 0.248(weight) (multiple regression)	
	Weight estimated from age = $\hat{w}$ (1)	actual weight − weight estimated from age = $w - \hat{w}$ (2)	SBP estimated from age = $\hat{SBP}$ (3)	Actual SBP − SBP estimated from age = $SBP - \hat{SBP}$ (4)	SBP estimated from age *and* weight = $\hat{SBP}'$ (5)	Actual SBP − SBP estimated from age and weight = $SBP - \hat{SBP}'$ (6)
1	172.4	−27.4	136.6	−4.6	129.8	2.2
2	185.5	30.5	144.4	10.6	152.0	3.0
3	178.0	−63.0	139.9	−9.9	124.3	5.7
4	166.8	3.2	133.2	8.8	134.0	8.0
5	187.4	−15.4	145.5	4.5	141.7	8.3
6	159.4	6.6	128.8	−0.8	130.4	−2.4
7	161.2	2.8	129.9	−3.9	130.6	−4.6
8	165.0	−13.0	132.1	−14.1	128.9	−10.9
9	185.5	89.5	144.4	35.6	166.6	13.4
10	178.0	43.0	139.9	−15.9	150.6	−26.6
11	159.4	15.6	128.8	21.2	132.7	17.3
12	187.4	−55.4	145.5	−11.5	131.8	2.2
13	185.5	2.5	144.4	−4.4	145.0	−5.0
14	185.5	−7.5	144.4	−2.4	142.5	−0.5
15	179.9	−11.9	141.1	−13.1	138.1	−10.1
Total	2636.9	0.1	2078.9	0.1	2079.0	0

variable and systolic blood pressure after removal of a component linearly related to age (column 4) as the dependent variable, we get

$$SBP - S\hat{B}P = 0.005 + 0.248(\text{weight} - \hat{\text{weight}})$$

The important point is that the coefficient of the weight discrepancy in this *simple* regression is identical to the coefficient for weight shown in the *multiple* regression equation at the top of columns 5 and 6 in Table 6-2.

ASSUMPTIONS UNDERLYING MULTIPLE REGRESSION METHODS

To simplify exposition, we summarize the assumptions underlying least-squares estimation of multiple regression parameters in terms of the specific model for two X variables:

$$Y = A + B_1 X_1 + B_2 X_2 + e \tag{6-7}$$

where A, B_1, and B_2 are population parameters, X_1, X_2, and Y are variables in the population, and e is the difference between the actual Y and that predicted by the model.

Assumptions Related to Model Fitting the Data

The first two assumptions to be made are

1. *Linearity*   For every pair of X_1 and X_2 values, the mean of the corresponding Y values lies on a flat surface.
2. *No interaction*   The effect of changes in X_1 on Y is independent of the level of X_2.

Both these assumptions relate to how well the model fits the sample data at hand. The basic method for testing whether they hold (at least approximately) is to examine the error in fit ($y_i - \hat{y}_i$) for various categories of observed values. Fitting the coefficients by the method of least squares will ensure that $\sum(y_i - \hat{y}_i) = 0$. The question of satisfactory fit relates to whether or not this sum is approximately zero for various subgroups of x values. Systematic errors suggest that the model is inadequate.

For example, suppose that observed x_1 values are grouped in quartiles and that corresponding $y_i - \hat{y}_i$ values are averaged for each quartile. There should be a similar average for each quartile of x_1. Also, $y_i - \hat{y}_i$ differences can be averaged in association with quartiles of all other x variables and with simple cross-classification of x variables. If, for example, the average value of $y_i - \hat{y}_i$ associated with x_1 and x_2 both high is much different from the average when x_1 is high and x_2 low, perhaps the model requires a term for interaction. All that follows in this text with respect to multivariate methods presumes that the model is a reasonably adequate description of the data in the sense that the mean values of the $y_i - \hat{y}_i$ discrepancies are approximately equal (i.e., not far from zero) for various subgroups. Thus, $\sum (y_i - \hat{y}_i)/n$ computed for each of several subgroups representing cross-classifications of the x variables reflects the extent to which the model fits the data within subgroups.

To illustrate this concept, we return to column 6 of Table 6-2, in which are shown $y_i - \hat{y}_i$ values calculated for each individual using a multiple linear regression model. (Table 6-2 uses the specific notation SBP-SBP̂ rather than $y_i - \hat{y}_i$.) As required by the model, the sum of these discrepancies over all individuals equals zero. However, this overall total of zero might be the consequence of large positive discrepancies in most subgroups balanced by very large negative discrepancies in a few others. Under those circumstances we are unlikely to consider the fit adequate.

To investigate this possibility we look at the average of the discrepancies between the model values and the actual values in four subgroups, as shown in Table 6-3. Recalling that actual systolic blood pressure values ranged from 118 to 180 and considering the substantive meaning of an average systolic blood pressure difference of 4 to 5 mm Hg, we can conclude that the model, in some sense, is similar to the data. Of course, to permit easy verification of the numbers, this trivial example is based on fewer cases than would be included in any real study. However, the principal point being made is that, in addition to appropriate tests of significance, you should look at the average agreement in major subsets of the data and, based on substantive considerations, make a judgment as to adequacy of fit.

At times, the observation of $\sum (y_i - \hat{y}_i)/n$ in various groups suggests ways of improving the model (e.g., adding cross-product terms, such as $x_1 x_2$, or squared terms, such as x_1^2), but if the end result shows one or more major subcategories of data with poor fit, the model is suspect.

Note that the preceding discussion deals exclusively with the extent of the discrepancy between model and data and not with any statistical significance testing to determine whether the decrease in residual error of, say, a four parameter model over, a three-parameter model is any greater than what could reasonably be expected by chance alone. This latter point is fully discussed in standard texts [54].

Table 6-3. Agreement Between Data and Prediction from Multiple Linear Regression Model in Four Age-Weight Sub-Classes (based on Tables 6-1 and 6-2)

Age	Weight	n	$\Sigma(\text{SBP} - \text{SBP}̂')/n$
< 53	< 172	6	−0.3
< 53	⩾ 172	2	−4.6
⩾ 53	< 172	2	−4.0
⩾ 53	⩾ 172	5	+3.8

Assumptions Related to Estimates of Variance and Significance Tests

Adding to our list of assumptions, we have

3. *Independence of observations*   Knowledge of the *Y* value for any individual provides no information about the *Y* value for any other individual.
4. *Homoscedasticity*   For every pair of X_1 and X_2 values, the variance of *Y* (var *e*) is a constant.
5. *Normality*   For every pair of X_1 and X_2 values, *Y* is normally distributed.

In epidemiologic studies, assumption 3 is almost always true. If variances are not constant as required by assumption 4, there are methods for weighting the observations so that coefficients and variances can be properly estimated. As the sample statistics b_1 and b_2 are essentially sums, their sampling distribution tends toward normality even when the *Y* values are not normally distributed as required by assumption 5.

It is beyond the scope of this book to provide the reader with the details of the calculation of least-squares regression coefficients, their estimated standard error, and the many other specifics required for data analysis. Epidemiologists require a general understanding of some multivariate methods, but most need statistical assistance in carrying out the specific analyses required by particular studies.

MULTIPLE REGRESSION FOR CATEGORICAL VARIABLES

Multiple regression methods for categorical data have been described by Feldstein [55]. They are analogous to directly standardized rates but include the possibility of adjusting for many variables at one time. We begin by assuming that *y* and all *x* variables are attributes, i.e., they have the value 1 if the attribute they represent is *present* and the value 0 if it is *absent*. If should be noted that measurement variables can be transformed to attributes, e.g., age < 45 = 0 and age $\geq$ 45 = 1. Thus, the method described here applies both to attributes and to measurement variables that have been transformed to attributes.

If we also assume that each *x* variable adds a constant amount to *y*, independent of other *x* values, the following model might suitably describe the relationship between y_j predicted and a set of x_i values:

$$\hat{y}_j = b_0 + b_1 x_{1j} + b_2 x_{2j} + b_3 x_{3j} \qquad (6\text{-}8)$$

For each individual, this does not make too much sense since all the *x* are either 1 or 0. However, after replacing *x* with the 1 and 0 values appropriate to each individual and then summing Equation 6-8 over all *n* individuals, we get:

$$\sum_{j=1}^{n} \hat{y}_j = nb_0 + b_1 \sum_{j=1}^{n} x_{ij} + b_2 \sum_{j=1}^{n} x_{2j} + b_3 \sum_{j=1}^{n} x_{3j}$$

If the b are determined by the method of least squares, then $\sum \hat{y}_j = \sum y_j$; that is, the sum of all predicted y_j values equals the sum of all actual y_j values. Substituting $\sum y_j$ for $\sum \hat{y}_j$ and dividing both sides of the equation by n, we get:

$$\bar{y} = b_0 + b_1\bar{x}_1 + b_2\bar{x}_2 + b_3\bar{x}_3 \tag{6-9}$$

At this point, it will simplify our discussion of multiple regression for categorical data if we assign to the variables in Equation 6-9 the following meanings from the Israeli Ischemic Heart Disease study sample data used previously:

$y = 1$ if myocardial infarction is present
$y = 0$ if myocardial infarction is absent
$x_1 = 1$ if SBP $\geqslant 140$
$x_1 = 0$ if SBP < 140
$x_2 = 1$ if the individual is age 40 through 49
$x_2 = 0$ if the individual is not age 40 through 49
$x_3 = 1$, if the individual is age 50 through 59
$x_3 = 0$ if the individual is not age 50 through 59

Recalling that data were presented for individuals age $\geqslant 60$ in the study sample, it may appear that we have neglected to assign a code to this age group, but we have in fact assigned such a code, however. The code for age $\geqslant 60$ is $x_2 = 0$ and $x_3 = 0$, i.e., not 40 to 49 and not 50 to 59. Binary data can be used in this way to code data classified into any number of groups. Because complications arise in solving the regression equations whenever they include perfectly correlated variables, it is necessary to code classification data using one fewer variable than the number of categories. To illustrate with blood pressure, two categories (SBP $\geqslant 140$ and SBP < 140) are coded into one variable, x_1, as shown above. The three age categories require two variables (x_2 and x_3). If we use another variable (x_4) to define age $\geqslant 60$, perfect correlation would exist, in that values for x_2 and x_3 would determine x_4. For example, if x_2 and x_3 were both 0, x_4 would necessarily $= 1$. This perfect correlation is exactly the type referred to above as interfering with the solution to the equations for regression coefficients. Since such a variable would cause trouble and provides no additional information, we avoid using it.

Returning to Equation 6-9 with variables as defined, $\bar{y}$ can be interpreted as the crude rate for myocardial infarction prevalence. We can modify this crude rate into various adjusted rates or differences between adjusted rates as follows. Suppose we use the least-squares regression coefficients to determine the prevalence rate for myocardial infarction *if* everyone in the population had SBP $\geq$ 140, with all other variables unchanged. This would mean that x_1 for every individual is 1 and that the summation of Equation 6-8 over all individuals divided by n would equal

$$\bar{y}_{\text{adj}} \text{ (if all SBP} \geq 140) = b_0 + b_1 + b_2 \bar{x}_2 + b_3 \bar{x}_3 \qquad (6\text{-}10)$$

This is identical to Equation 6-9 except that $b_1 \bar{x}_1$ has been changed to b_1 (with each individual having $x_1 = 1$, the sum of $b_1 x_1$ over all n individuals equals nb_1 and dividing this by n gives b_1). The $\bar{y}_{\text{adj}}$ of Equation 6-10 could be compared with another $\bar{y}_{\text{adj}}$ in which everyone had SBP < 140 but was otherwise unchanged. The adjusted prevalence rate for SBP < 140 requires that all values of x_1 equal zero. Summing the value of $b_1 \times 0$ over all individuals and dividing by n results, of course, in zero. Thus, the adjusted prevalence for SBP < 140 is

$$\bar{y}_{\text{adj}} \text{ (if all SBP} < 140) = b_0 + 0 + b_2 \bar{x}_2 + b_3 \bar{x}_3 \qquad (6\text{-}11)$$

Note that the difference between adjusted rates for those with SBP $\geq$ 140 and SBP < 140 is exactly b_1 and that the effect of possible age differences between those with higher SBP and lower SBP has been eliminated by using the identical age distribution in the estimation of both adjusted rates.

Thus b_1 is the difference between prevalence rates for myocardial infarction comparing SBP $\geq$ 140 ($x_1 = 1$) with SBP < 140 ($x_1 = 0$), adjusted for possible age differences between those with higher or lower blood pressure. In general, b_i may be interpreted as the difference in adjusted rates comparing persons for whom $x_i = 1$ with persons in the reference class for that variable. For dichotomous variables, the reference class is represented by those for whom $x = 0$. For the age variable with three categories, the reference class is represented by those individuals age $\geq$ 60 who are included in the equation not explicitly but only indirectly through x_2 and x_3. Those who are *not* 40 to 49 and *not* 50 to 59, i.e., $x_2 = 0$ *and* $x_3 = 0$, are in the reference class for age. Thus in Equation 6-9, b_2 is the difference in MI prevalence between those 40 to 49 and those 60 and over, adjusted for SBP differences between the two age groups. Similarly, b_3 is the difference in MI prevalence between those 50 to 59 and those 60 and over, adjusted for possible SBP differences between the two groups.

Should we wish to compare adjusted rates for those age 40 to 49 ($x_2 = 1$) and those age 50 to 59 ($x_3 = 1$), i.e., a comparison not involving the reference class age 60 to 69 ($x_2 = 0$ *and* $x_3 = 0$), only $b_2 - b_3$ need be computed. Since b_2 is the difference between age 40 to 49 and the reference age and b_3 is the difference between age 50 to 59 and the reference age, $b_2 - b_3$ is the difference in adjusted rates between age 40 to 49 and age 50 to 59.

To compute adjusted rates for *any class of a specific variable* (i.e., assuming everyone in the population belongs to that class but all other variables are unchanged), we must add to the crude rate the regression coefficient for that class minus $(\sum_i b_i \sum_j x_{ij})/n$, with the summation over index j extending over all n individuals in the regression analysis and the sum over i extending over all classes *of the specific variable*. We illustrate this by computing an adjusted rate for persons age 40 to 49. This is the MI prevalence rate that would exist if the binary regression model were applicable to the data and if all persons were age 40 to 49 ($x_2 = 1$) with SBP values unchanged. Returning to Equation 6-9 this is

$$
\begin{array}{ll}
b_0 + b_1\bar{x}_1 + b_2 & \text{adjusted rate if all were age 40 to 49} \\
b_0 + b_1\bar{x}_1 + b_2\bar{x}_2 + b_3\bar{x}_3 & \text{crude rate, all ages as given} \\
\hline
b_2 - b_2\bar{x}_2 - b_3\bar{x}_3 & \text{excess of adjusted rate over crude rate}
\end{array}
$$

which equals

$$
b_2 - \frac{1}{n}\sum_{i=2}^{3} b_i \sum_{j=1}^{n} x_{ij}
$$

with summation of the index i over the two variables used to define age class, x_2 and x_3.

To compute the difference between the crude and adjusted rates for persons in the reference class, age 60 to 69, we have

$$
\begin{array}{ll}
b_0 + b_1\bar{x}_1 & \text{adjusted rate if all were age 60 to 69} \\
b_0 + b_1\bar{x}_1 + b_2\bar{x}_2 + b_3\bar{x}_3 & \text{crude rate, all ages as given} \\
\hline
0 - b_2\bar{x}_2 - b_3\bar{x}_3 & \text{excess of adjusted rate over crude rate}
\end{array}
$$

The difference between adjusted and crude rates, as stated above, is the regression coefficient for the adjusted class minus $(b_i \sum_{j=1}^{n} x_{ij})/n$ summed over all classes of the variable to which the adjusted class belongs.

When the adjusted class is the reference class, we take its regression coefficient to be zero.

To review, the adjusted rate for age 40 to 49 exceeds the crude rate by $b_2 - b_2\bar{x}_2 - b_3\bar{x}_3$, and the adjusted rate for the reference category, age $\geqslant 60$, exceeds the crude rate by $0 - b_2\bar{x}_2 - b_3\bar{x}_3$. Thus, the amount by which the adjusted rate for age 40 to 49 exceeds the adjusted rate for the reference category is b_2, the regression coefficient for age 40 to 49 (x_2).

As described above, adjusted rates can be calculated for any binary variable in relation to its reference class. This can be done whether the other variables are binary or continuous. If x_1, the variable for SBP in the preceding example, were a continuous variable, the difference in MI prevalence rates between age 40 to 49 and age 60 to 69, adjusted so that the difference in prevalence rates is un-affected by blood pressure differences, would still be exactly equal to b_2. Although the special computational convenience of having differences in adjusted rates represented by regression coefficients applies only to variables expressed in binary form, in other respects multiple regression using continuous variables and binary multiple regression are alike. In either case, the regression coefficient b_i represents the average change in y associated with a unit change in x_i, after adjusting for the linear relationships between all other x variables and x_i and between all other x variables and y. If x_i is a binary variable, then a unit change in x_i represents a change from x_i present to x_i absent (or vice versa). If x_i is a continuous variable, then a unit change in x_i may represent only 1 mmHg of blood pressure or 1 mg % of serum cholesterol, etc. No matter how x_i is expressed, however, b_i represents the average change in y associated with a unit change in x_i, adjusted for all other x variables included in the regression.

An advantage of the categorization approach is that it avoids assuming any particular form of regression for the variable categorized. For example, if age is categorized into three classes, the middle class coefficient may indicate that middle age adds, on the average, .15 to the rate for the young but the coefficient for the older class may indicate that older age adds nothing to the rate for the young.

DISCRIMINANT FUNCTIONS

Related to multiple linear regression but derived differently is the linear discriminant function. Given two groups, for example, sick (s) and well (w), with several x variables measured in each, we might wish to use the x variables to discriminate between the two groups. For each individual in each group we could form a score $z = b_1 x_1 + b_2 x_2 + b_3 x_3 + \ldots$

The b values would be the same for every individual in the two groups and would provide a weighted sum of the x values. If more weight is given to those x variables that discriminate well and less weight to those that discriminate poorly, we have a discriminant function. Fisher solved this problem [56] by finding the b values that maximize the function

$$\frac{|\bar{z}_s - \bar{z}_w|}{\text{var}(\bar{z}_s - \bar{z}_w)} \tag{6-12}$$

where $\bar{z}_s$ is the average value of $\sum b_i x_i$ in the sick population and $\bar{z}_w$ its average value in the well population. By choosing the b values that made the difference in average scores as large as possible in relation to the variance of the difference, Fisher obtained the linear discriminant function.

Discrimination using the x variables is generally accomplished by designating some value of z as a separation point, with individuals having values that large or larger classified as belonging to one population and all those with smaller z values classified as belonging to the other population. Obviously, the error in the first classification can be made as small as desired. Simply designate all individuals having the smallest z score obtained, or larger, as members of the sick population. Not a single member of the actual sick population would be missed by this classification rule. However, none of the well individuals would have scores below this cutoff point and the error in classifying well persons would be 100 percent. If the two populations are multivariate normal with the same variance-covariance matrix for any specific size of error in classifying one category, the discriminant function minimizes the error classifying the other category.

Epidemiologists are usually less interested in actual discrimination between two populations than in interpreting the discriminant function coefficients, e.g., for evaluating the importance of risk factors. Knowledge of the fact that discriminant function coefficients are essentially similar to multiple regression coefficients is helpful in this regard. If the identical data set (with y as a binary variable) is tabulated to obtain multiple regression coefficients a, b_1, b_2, b_3, etc., and also to obtain discriminant function coefficients which, for convenience, we label $\beta_1, \beta_2, \beta_3$, etc., then the ratio of any two discriminant function coefficients β_i/β_j is exactly equal to the b_i/b_j ratio of the corresponding regression coefficients. This equality shows that discriminant function coefficients reflect the relationship between a particular x variable and y after adjustment for all other variables, as discussed earlier for multiple regression coefficients.

This presentation of multiple regression, including binary variable multiple regression and discriminant functions, is intended to provide some general understanding of these procedures. Techniques for computing coefficients, their estimated standard error, and related matters are outside the scope of this book, and statistical assistance regarding them is recommended [1,5,54].

MULTIPLE LOGISTIC FUNCTIONS

Whenever y is a binary variable, nothing in the method of multiple regression prevents an estimate of y from being less than zero or more than unity. Since the estimated value of y is not defined as a probability, values outside the 0 to 1 range are not impossible or wrong, but neither are they entirely satisfactory as an estimate of a variable that equals zero if the condition is absent and unity if it is present. Although this is an undesirable feature of multiple regression methods applied to dependent binary variables (y), it does not invalidate the method. The key to the usefulness of multiple regression methods is whether the model fits the data. Nevertheless, it clearly would be an improvement in interpreting regression coefficients if estimates of y (when it is a binary variable) could be expressed as probabilities.

This, in addition to other benefits in analysis and interpretation, results if the data are fitted to a multiple logistic function. This function was first used by

Cornfield et al. [57] as an estimator of risk when the joint distribution of all the independent variables was multivariate normal with the same variance-covariance matrix for both sick and well populations. For two x variables, the function has the form

$$\hat{y} = \frac{1}{1 + e^{-(\alpha + \beta_1 x_1 + \beta_2 x_2)}} \tag{6-13}$$

Cornfield used this function to estimate the risk of developing coronary heart disease (y) from a knowledge of systolic blood pressure (x_1) and serum cholesterol (x_2). By logarithmic transformation of x_1 and x_2, approximate bivariate normality was achieved for the joint distribution of x_1 and x_2 separately among those developing and those not developing heart disease. The transformed variables also demonstrated approximate equality of the two variance-covariance matrices. The approximately bivariate normal distribution for these two groups is as shown in Figure 6-1, where the height of the

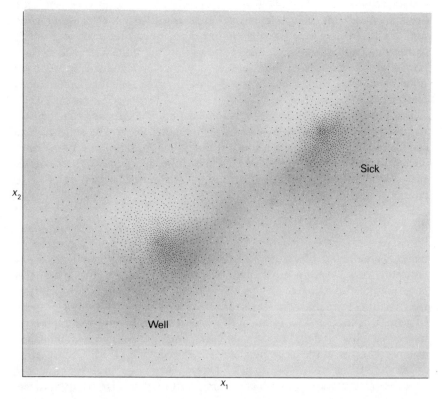

Figure 6-1. Number of persons at each x_1, x_2 point in sick and well populations. Number is indicated as a third dimension rising vertically from the plane of the page.

distribution above the paper at any "point" represents the number of individuals in the distribution having x_1 and x_2 values intersecting at that point. Although it is not possible to show this clearly in the diagram because both joint distributions are bivariate normal (i.e., for every value of x_1, x_2 is normally distributed and vice versa), all points within the range of x_1 and x_2 values shown in the figure have some representation from each distribution. The risk of developing heart disease for an individual with a specific x_1 and x_2 value can then be expressed as the number in the sick distribution at point x_1, x_2 divided by the total number in both distributions at point x_1, x_2. This total equals the number in the sick distribution at point x_1, x_2 plus the number in the well distribution at point x_1, x_2. With this basic definition of risk and with x variables transformed, if necessary, so that they are multivariate normal, the multiple logistic function results as an estimator of risk. If the distributions are bivariate normal (or, in the case of three or more x variables, multivariate normal), it is not a difficult matter to calculate the height of the distribution for any particular joint value of x_1 and x_2. Clearly, this height of the distribution (called the ordinate) is a function of x_1 and x_2 and of the parameters of the two distributions. As reported by Cornfield et al. [57], for relating systolic blood pressure and cholesterol to risk, the parameters for each population, sick and well, are the mean and variance of systolic blood pressure and serum cholesterol, the correlation coefficient between them, and the size of each population. The result obtained by finding the height of each distribution at point x_1, x_2 and dividing the height of the sick distribution by the sum of the heights of the two distributions is what would be obtained from the logistic function shown as Equation 6-13, where α, β_1, and β_2 are functions of the parameters of the two distributions. Since in the general multivariate case, the coefficients of the multiple logistic function require matrix algebra for their complete description, we shall refer to them only as values computable from the number of cases, the mean values and variances of the x_i, and the covariances of the x_i and x_j for each distribution.

It is interesting to note that β_1 and β_2 are exactly equal to the linear discriminant function coefficients that would have resulted from relating x_1 and x_2 to binary y in a linear discriminant function analysis. The parameter α has no parallel in the discriminant analysis and is related to the general level of risk. Particular values of $\sum \beta_i x_i$ for specific individuals raise or lower that general level. The discriminant scores, on the other hand, have no intrinsic meaning as to risk or anything else. Their only interpretation is with reference to being larger or smaller than other scores in the study. Individuals with the largest scores are judged to belong to one group and those with the smallest scores to another.

Cornfield's original derivation of the logistic function as an estimator of risk depended on multivariate normality of the x variables within both sick and well populations, together with equal variances and covariances in the two populations. This latter point is necessary or else the logistic function would have to contain terms involving products of x variables such as $\beta_3 x_1 x_2$. The need for product terms to obtain a satisfactory fit between model and data suggests the presence of interaction. In practice, logistic functions are usually calculated without these product terms and the terms are added only if the model fits the data significantly better with their addition. Of course, whenever a priori knowledge points to the presence of interaction between variables, product terms should be included.

Because this function is one that increases only with increasing values of $\alpha + \sum \beta_i x_i$, we can demonstrate that the y_i values computed from the logistic function have the property required of probabilities. To show that they are limited to the range zero to unity inclusive, we can substitute $+\infty$ and $-\infty$ for $\alpha + \sum \beta_i x_i$ in Equation 6-13. Since $\alpha + \sum \beta_i x_i$ cannot be larger or smaller than these limits, the resultant values of the function are

for $\alpha + \sum \beta_i x_i = +\infty$:

$$\hat{y} = \frac{1}{1 + e^{-\infty}} = \frac{1}{1 + 0} = 1$$

for $\alpha + \sum \beta_i x_i = -\infty$:

$$\hat{y} = \frac{1}{1 + e^{\infty}} = 0$$

To complement these calculations, we also solve for $\hat{y}$ if $\alpha + \sum \beta_i x_i = 0$. In that case,

$$\hat{y} = \frac{1}{1 + e^{-0}} = \frac{1}{1 + 1} = \frac{1}{2}$$

Thus, if the exponent of e is very large and positive the risk is close to unity, if the exponent of e is zero the risk is $\frac{1}{2}$, and if the exponent of e is very large and negative the risk is close to zero.

Up to this point, the multiple logistic function has been derived from the multivariate normal distribution of the x variables in both sick and well populations. However, the real world is rarely multivariate normal, nor is it always possible to transform variables so that multivariate normality results. For example, binary variables cannot possibly be transformed to normal. Nevertheless, it has been found that the logistic function fits the data in a variety of circumstances in which the distribution of the x variables is surely not multivariate normal [58–60]. The fit of the logistic function to the data can be assessed rather simply in accord with the principles* outlined earlier in this chapter and illustrated in the following procedure for a function with three x variables.

1. Calculate $\hat{y}_j$ for each individual in the study by using α and the β_1, β_2, and β_3 values from the multiple logistic function for every individual, together with the specific values of x_1, x_2, and x_3 relevant to each individual.

Table 6-4. Evaluating Fit of Multiple Logistic Risk Function to Data by Comparing Diabetes Cases Observed with Cases Predicted by Risk Function [60]

	Diabetes incidence cases	
Percentile of risk function array	Number observed (Σy_j)	Number expected according to multiple logistic risk function $(\Sigma \hat{y}_j)$
0–24	10	10.5
25–49	23	19.5
50–74	28	31.3
75–100	70	72.1

2. Array the $\hat{y}_j$ values in order of size.
3. Divide the array of step 2 into quartiles, quintiles, deciles, or some other grouping.
4. Add up the $\hat{y}_j$ values within each group and compare the sum with the sum of the actual y_j values in that group. The sum of the $\hat{y}_j$ equals the number of cases expected according to the model, and the sum of the y_j equals the number of cases actually observed.

For technical reasons these observed and expected values cannot always be summarized ($\sum[(O - E)^2/E]$) into the ordinary goodness-of-fit χ^2 value [61], but a good sense of agreement or lack of it can usually be obtained by inspection. An illustration of this procedure for checking fit using data from Kahn et al. [60] is shown as Table 6-4. In this instance the $\hat{y}_j$ values (probability of becoming diabetic) were arrayed in order from smallest to largest and then grouped into quartiles. The agreement between observed cases and expected cases (i.e., the sum of the probabilities of becoming a case) is quite satisfactory.

The observation that the multiple logistic risk function often fits rather well to data that are obviously not normal has an explanation. Although the distribution of the x variables in multivariate normal fashion is sufficient to define risk according to the multiple logistic function, it is not necessary. Univariate normality of the sum $\alpha + \sum \beta_i x_i$ also leads to definition of risk according to the multiple logistic function [58].

An alternative approach with respect to the multiple logistic function is to assume that the risk function is multiple logistic and to determine the coefficients by methods analogous to the least-squares fit of a nonlinear function [62]. The assumption that multiple logistic is the correct form of the risk function is in some way equivalent to the assumptions about the form of the multivariate distribution of the x variables. The least-squares regression approach does lead to different estimates of the coefficients, although these are frequently quite similar to the discriminant approach [59,60]. If the distribution of the x variables is multivariate normal, the logistic function with β coefficients equal to discriminant coefficients correctly defines risk. If the logistic function is assumed as the correct representation of risk, then the coefficients are calculated as in nonlinear regression and thus require more computer time and memory storage than does the calculation of the discriminant function coefficients. At present, a consensus favors the nonlinear regression approach as being more correct. My advice is to use the simpler and cheaper discriminant approach for exploratory tabulations and the more expensive regression calculations for material to be published. As computers develop increasing speed and greater storage memory, the cost difference between the two approaches will decrease, and I would then accept the consensus favoring the regression approach without qualification. One final comment: if the use of discriminant coefficients results in a very good agreement between $\sum \hat{y}_j$ and $\sum y_j$ in the several groups (deciles, quartiles, etc.) for which it is computed, the nonlinear regression coefficients will probably not differ much from the discriminant coefficients.

In addition to providing an estimate of y_j that is interpretable as a probability, another desirable feature of the multiple logistic function is that each of the β_i can be interpreted as the logarithm of an odds ratio relating disease to the variable x_i, after adjustment for all other x variables. We demonstrate this first for a binary variable, $x_1 = 1$ or 0, in a function with three x variables:

$$\hat{y} = \text{estimated probability of event} = 1/(1 + e^{-(\alpha + \beta_1 x_1 + \beta_2 x_2 + \beta_3 x_3)})$$

$$1 - \hat{y} = \text{estimated probability of no event}$$

$$= 1 - [1/(1 + e^{-(\alpha + \beta_1 x_1 + \beta_2 x_2 + \beta_3 x_3)})]$$

$$= \frac{1 + e^{-(\alpha + \beta_1 x_1 + \beta_2 x_2 + \beta_3 x_3)}}{1 + e^{-(\alpha + \beta_1 x_1 + \beta_2 x_2 + \beta_3 x_3)}} - \frac{1}{1 + e^{-(\alpha + \beta_1 x_1 + \beta_2 x_2 + \beta_3 x_3)}}$$

$$= \frac{e^{-(\alpha + \beta_1 x_1 + \beta_2 x_2 + \beta_3 x_3)}}{1 + e^{-(\alpha + \beta_1 x_1 + \beta_2 x_2 + \beta_3 x_3)}}$$

By dividing the probability of an event by the probability of no event, we get the odds of the event. To illustrate this with numeric data, suppose that the probability of an event is 3 out of 10 and the probability of its not happening is 7 out of 10. If we divide the probability of occurrence (3/10) by the probability of nonoccurrence (7/10), we get 3/7. This is the odds that the event will occur. Returning to the logistic function, the estimated odds of an event are

$$\frac{\hat{y}}{1 - \hat{y}} = \frac{1}{e^{-(\alpha + \beta_1 x_1 + \beta_2 x_2 + \beta_3 x_3)}} = e^{\alpha + \beta_1 x_1 + \beta_2 x_2 + \beta_3 x_3} \qquad (6\text{-}14)$$

The relative odds of an event (odds ratio), which compares those for whom x_1 is present ($x_1 = 1$) with those for whom x_1 is absent ($x_1 = 0$) is

$$\text{odds ratio} = \frac{e^{\alpha + \beta_1 + \beta_2 x_2 + \beta_3 x_3}}{e^{(\alpha + 0 + \beta_2 x_2 + \beta_3 x_3)}}$$

$$= e^{(\alpha + \beta_1 + \beta_2 x_2 + \beta_3 x_3) - (\alpha + 0 + \beta_2 x_2 + \beta_3 x_3)}$$

$$= e^{\beta_1}$$

Thus,

$$\ln \text{ odds ratio} = \beta_1 \qquad (6\text{-}15)$$

If, for example, x_1 relates to the presence or absence of diabetes and y to the probability of developing a myocardial infarction, then e^{β_1}, the antilog of β_1, provides the ratio of odds of myocardial infarction for those with diabetes present to the odds for those with diabetes absent. As in the case of multiple linear regression, β_1 is adjusted for linear association with other x variables. However, keep in mind that the function $\alpha + \beta_1 x_1 + \beta_2 x_2 + \beta_3 x_3$ is linear not in probabilities but in the natural logarithm of the odds that an event will occur.

To illustrate the essential equivalence between adjusted odds ratios computed using the multiple logistic function and those computed using the M-H procedure, we refer to Table 6-5. These data are from a study of serologic markers of hepatitis B among Italian navy recruits. Only two of the nine variables in Table 6-5 show adjusted odds ratio differences of any consequence. These are region of residence, 1.67 versus 1.42, and multiple injection scars, 3.51 versus 2.99. In each of these instances, the odds ratio derived from multiple logistic analysis is larger. The fit of the data to the logistic model, determined as in Table 6-4, is entirely satisfactory. However, failure to find a difference between the actual data and the data predicted by a model does not, of course, establish the model as correct, and the calculation of the multiple logistic coefficients depends upon the correctness of the model as a reflection of risk. The M-H calculation, however, depends upon nothing. Thus, when the two methods differ for equivalent calculations (i.e., all variables are attributes), I would choose the M-H result. When they are not different, as in seven of nine instances in Table 6-5, the comparison is a valuable reenforcement of the findings and a useful check on all aspects of the computations. When a method is as simple and free of assumptions as the M-H procedure, it deserves to receive a strong recommendation, and I do not hesitate to give it.

Returning to the multiple logistic function, if x_1 were a continuous variable, the derivation shown above for x_1 as a binary variable would lead to β_1 as the natural logarithm of the odds ratio relating the odds of developing the disease to a one-unit increase in x_1 (e.g., comparing $x_1 = 150$ to $x_1 = 149$). If we wanted an odds ratio related to a 10- or 20-unit increase in x_1, we would begin the derivation with Equation 6-14:

$$\text{odds of event to no event} = e^{\alpha + \beta_1 x_1 + \beta_2 x_2 + \beta_3 x_3}$$

Table 6-5. Adjusted Odds Ratios for Presence of Serologic Markers of Hepatitis B Among Italian Nary Recruits[a]

Variable	Adjustment by multiple logistic analysis[b]	Adjustment by M-H procedure
Age ($> 19 / \leqslant 19$)	.77	.79
Number of siblings ($> 3 / \leqslant 3$)	1.58	1.62
Region of birth $\left(\dfrac{\text{southern Italy or islands}}{\text{northern or central Italy}}\right)$	1.50	1.40
Region of residence $\left(\dfrac{\text{southern Italy or islands}}{\text{northern or central Italy}}\right)$	1.67	1.42
Education level (above elementary/elementary)	.62	.62
Altitude of residence $\left(\dfrac{\text{hills or mountains}}{\text{lowlands}}\right)$	.77	.78
History of jaundice (yes/no)	1.71	1.66
History of intravenous injection (yes/no)	1.45	1.47
Multiple injection scars noted (yes/no)	3.51	2.99

[a] The odds ratio for each variable is adjusted for possible confounding by all other variables in the table.
[b] No assumption of multivariate normality among those with and without positive serologic markers of hepatitis B. Coefficients estimated by methods similar to those described in Walker and Duncan [62].
Source: Unpublished data from the Merck Sharp and Dohme Epidemiologic Research Center, Rome, Italy.

odds ratio comparing those with $x_1 = K + 10$ to those with $x_1 = K$

$$= \frac{e^{\alpha + \beta_1(10 + K) + \beta_2 x_2 + \beta_3 x_3}}{e^{\alpha + \beta_1 K + \beta_2 x_2 + \beta_3 x_3}}$$

$$= e^{\alpha + 10\beta_1 + \beta_1 K + \beta_2 x_2 + \beta_3 x_3 - (\alpha + \beta_1 K + \beta_2 x_2 + \beta_3 x_3)}$$

$$= e^{10\beta_1}$$

$$\text{ln odds ratio} = 10\beta_1$$

Thus, we see that the natural logarithm of the odds ratio comparing two different values of x_1 equals β_1 multiplied by the difference in those x_1 values.

In all cases, the natural logarithm of the odds ratio (β_i) relating x_i to odds of disease has been adjusted for linear relationships as discussed in the section on multiple linear regression. Although the multiple logistic function coefficients are nonlinear with respect to *probability* of risk, the *ln odds* equation is exactly analogous to multiple linear regression:

$$\text{ln odds} = \ln\left(\frac{\hat{y}}{1 - \hat{y}}\right) = \alpha + \beta_1 x_1 + \beta_2 x_2 + \beta_3 x_3 \qquad (6\text{-}16)$$

Often there is interest in knowing which of the x variables has the most effect on risk (y). This is a distinctly different question from which x variable is the most "significant" (i.e., most unusual under the null hypothesis). The largest β_i in terms of absolute value (disregarding sign) is not necessarily the one with the most effect, since the size of β_i depends on the units of x_i. If x_i is weight, it might be measured in grams or in kilograms. The β_i for x_i measured in kilograms would be 1000 times larger than the β_i for x_i measured in grams. Obviously, then, the largest β_i is in part determined by the accident of choice of units. A simple procedure permitting comparison of how β_i values affect y, free of distortion due to differences in units, is to compare $\beta_i \sigma_i$ values. Note first that σ_i refers to the standard deviation of the x_i values. It is *not* the standard error of β_i that is wanted here but something that will remove the effect of arbitrary choice of units. Analogous to our previous derivation of $10\beta_1$ as the natural logarithm of the odds ratio comparing those with an x_1 value of $K + 10$ with those with an x_1 value of K, $\beta_i \sigma_i$ represents the natural logarithm of the odds ratio related to one standard deviation change in x_i. If x_i is a weight variable measured in grams, β_i would be $1/1000$ as large and σ_i would be 1000 times as large than the comparable values for x_i measured in kilograms. Thus, $\beta_i \sigma_i$ is independent of the choice of units and comparing $\beta_1 \sigma_1$ with $\beta_2 \sigma_2$, etc., to find the largest absolute value is an excellent way of determining which x variable has the most effect on the natural logarithm of the odds ratio.

The multiple logistic function can be used for relating x variables to prevalence of existing disease [63] and even for investigating difference in exposure between cases and controls in a retrospective study [63,64]. In the latter case, it should be obvious that α has no intrinsic meaning since the general level of risk in a case-control study is arbitrarily determined by the selected number of controls per case. Matched pair data can also be analyzed this way provided no meaning is attached to the β_i for those variables that are matched if they are represented in the function. The β_i for variables not matched should be interpreted as adjusted for association with all matched variables as well as all other variables in the study. The nature of the adjustment for *matched* variables is not limited, as previously outlined, to linear relationships but is more comprehensive.

There is a method of applying multiple logistic procedures to matched pair case-control data that emphasizes the paired data [65]. In this method, the y variable is the *difference* in disease status between case and control. This is always $1 - 0 = 1$. Similarly, each x variable for each pair is the difference between case and control for that variable.

Although it is certainly a valuable tool, multiple logistic analysis is unlikely to identify a different set of variables, as related to outcome, than would be identified by multiple linear regression. An example of this similarity can be found in a report on the Coronary Drug Project in which the data were analyzed by both methods [66].

CONSTRUCTION OF STRATA USING A MULTIVARIATE FUNCTION

Epidemiologists generally encounter multivariate methods used directly to reduce or eliminate confounding. However, such methods may also be used to establish strata within which the association of prime interest can be examined essentially free of confounding [67]. We can illustrate this approach by first assuming that we have the necessary data and have calculated a discriminant function relating age, blood pressure, serum cholesterol, cigarette smoking, and abdominal skinfold to the risk of myocardial infarction in men. Although it is somewhat artificial to consider one of these variables as the one of major interest and the others as just potential confounders, such considerations do arise. For the moment, imagine that we want to investigate the association of abdominal skinfold with risk of myocardial infarction free of possible confounding by the other variables. After calculating discriminant function coefficients for abdominal skinfold and for each of the other variables in the usual way, we do not compute the ordinary discriminant function score for each individual. Instead we compute a discriminant function score for each individual after fixing the abdominal skinfold coefficient at zero. The resultant scores represent the tendency of each individual to a higher or lower score with respect to development of myocardial infarction based solely on the potential confounding variables. These scores can, for example, be divided into quartiles, and then within each quartile the relationship of skinfold to myocardial infarction risk could be studied. The persons in each quartile would be roughly homogeneous as to myocardial infarction risk related to the non-skinfold variables, at least insofar as a linear combination of the potential confounders is able to discriminate risk. Thus comparisons in myocardial infarction risk between those with large abdominal skinfolds and those lacking this particular badge of overeating are free of the confounding that might result because those with large skinfolds tend to smoke more, have higher blood pressure, etc.

If skinfold is dichotomized within each quartile, we could summarize the relevant data in a 2 × 2 table. The individual 2 × 2 tables could then be combined by means of the Mantel-Haenszel procedure [47].

The use of the discriminant function is not essential for this procedure. Multiple linear regression or multiple logistic functions serve equally well. Remember, however, that multivariate functions used this way are not exempt from the basic requirement that they fit the data.

NOTE

* Selecting these with high, medium, or low risk under the model is equivalent to selecting the cross-classification categories for which risk is high, medium, or low.

7
Longitudinal Studies: Life Tables

The remark attributed to John Maynard Keynes that "in the long run we are all dead" [68] indicates why it is often insufficient to compare percentage mortality among those given treatment A with percentage mortality among those given treatment B. Obviously, if the period for observation of mortality is very long, Lord Keynes' dictum can be controlling. Forty years after a middle-aged or elderly population is treated, there can be little distinction in percentage dead among those given one treatment or another. Shorter investigations can avoid the more obvious consequences of our common mortality. Whether the investigation covers a long period or a short one, however, the difference between dying one year and dying ten years after treatment is of great importance not only to the individual survivor but to the epidemiologic analyst wishing to evaluate the two treatments.

The types of studies encountered by epidemiologists in which these problems arise include randomized, controlled clinical trials with moderately long to long observation time after treatment [69]; evaluation of differential mortality in different population groups, such as smokers and non-smokers [70]; summarization of mortality risk for groups, such as radiologists, hypothesized to be at greater than average risk [71]; and evaluation of survival after the diagnosis of specific types of cancer [72]. In all of these investigations, the end point is not necessarily mortality; it may be onset of disease or disability, for example, in accordance with study interests and objectives.

COMPUTATIONS AND ASSUMPTIONS

If longitudinal studies include data on persons observed for long periods or for varying lengths of time, some systematic procedure is required for summarizing the observations. The life table [73,74] provides one way of

Table 7-1. Basic Data Summarization for Survival After Cardiac Transplant

Postoperative interval (months)	Under observation at start of interval	Died during interval
0– 1.99	300	195
2– 3.99	105	27
4– 5.99	78	15
6– 7.99	63	12
8– 9.99	51	9
10–11.99	42	12
12–13.99	30	

handling such data, and we begin by describing a simple example. Assume that 300 persons have received cardiac transplants and that we wish to estimate the probability of surviving the surgery by one year. The data might be as shown in Table 7-1. The probability of dying during each interval is the number dying in the interval divided by the number alive at the beginning of the interval. More precisely, this quotient is the probability of dying during an interval for those alive at its beginning. Standard notation for this probability is $_nq_x$, read as "the probability of dying during the interval x to $x + n$ for those alive at time x." Other useful symbols are

x time at beginning of interval
O_x number under observation at exact time x
n length of interval
$_nd_x$ number dying in interval x to $x + n$
$_np_x$ probability of surviving from time x to time $x + n = 1 - {_nq_x}$

Table 7-2 restates the data from Table 7-1, incorporating the above notation and also columns for $_2q_x$ and $_2p_x$. Although n(equal to 2) is constant in this example, it does not have to be.

Table 7-2. Data from Table 7-1 with Life Table Calculations and Notation

Time at beginning of interval (months)	Under observation at time x	Died during interval	Probability of Dying during interval	Probability of Surviving through interval
x	O_x	$_2d_x$	$_2q_x$	$_2p_x$
0	300	195	.65	.35
2	105	27	.26	.74
4	78	15	.19	.81
6	63	12	19	.81
8	51	9	.18	.82
10	42	12	.29	.71
12	30			

Usually, the primary interest in data of this type is not in the probability of surviving through any particular interval but in the probability of surviving 6 months or 12 months or some other specific period from time 0, the time of surgery. To symbolize this cumulative, or overall, survival spanning several periods, we use a slightly different notation: $_nP_x$ symbolizes the probability of surviving from time x to time $x + n$ with the capital letter P signifying a period longer than a single interval. The $_nP_x$ is derived from the product of several $_np_x$ values as outlined below.

Suppose we wish to estimate the 12-month probability of survival after surgery. Obviously, to survive for 12 months one must survive the 2-month period beginning with $x = 0$ *and* the period beginning with $x = 2$ *and* the period beginning with $x = 4$ *and* . . . . Using notation analogous to the summation notation reviewed in Chapter 1 but with Π to represent the product of terms, we have*

$$_{12}P_0 = \prod_{i=0}^{5} {_2p_{2i}} = (_2p_0)(_2p_2)(_2p_4)(_2p_6)(_2p_8)(_2p_{10})$$

For the data in Table 7-2, this is

$$_{12}P_0 = (.35)(.74)(.81)(.81)(.82)(.71) = .10$$

The probability of surviving 12 months from the date of cardiac transplant (.10) corresponds to the number surviving to that date (30) divided by the number receiving transplants (300). Why, then, do we bother with the product of probabilities for surviving several periods when the desired statistic seems readily at hand, i.e., the number surviving to 12 months divided by the number given transplants? We do this because the number surviving to the time we wish to evaluate is almost always affected by cases withdrawn from the study or lost to observation before the evaluation time is reached. In Table 7-2, there happened to be no withdrawals or cases lost to observation and so the simple calculation is satisfactory.

The term *withdrawals* is used to describe persons still alive who must be dropped from a study because the length of time they have been in the study is shorter than the interval for which survival is being calculated. For example, in a calculation of five-year survival, someone who received initial treatment (and entered the study) three and a half years ago and was a survivor would have to be withdrawn before the start of the 4–4.99-year interval.

To illustrate how withdrawals come about, let us consider a survival study following a specific type of surgery for breast cancer. The study begins on January 1, 1970, and the data are analyzed as of December 31, 1978, using all information collected to that date. A woman treated on January 1, 1970, might contribute to data on survival from the seventh year after treatment to the eighth anniversary. However, a woman treated on July 1, 1975, and added to the study on that date cannot possibly provide any information about survival from the seventh to the eighth year after treatment. If the person treated on July 1, 1975, has survived until December 31, 1978, she must be treated as a subject who has been withdrawn during the fourth year of observation. For this individual, year 1 runs from July 1, 1975, to June 30, 1976, year 2 from July 1, 1976 to June 30, 1977, year 3 from July 1, 1977 to June 30, 1978, and year 4 from July 1, 1978 to June 30, 1979. However, since the study cutoff date is December 31, 1978, it is impossible for her to complete the fourth year of observation before the cutoff. If she has survived to the cutoff date, she must be withdrawn in the year that includes it.

Cases lost to observation are also considered as having been withdrawn alive, but the reason for their withdrawal is that the follow-up procedures failed to determine their status rather than that they had reached the limits of time for observation. Because withdrawals and losses to observation can have different effects on the estimated probability of survival, we use distinct terminology for them. We shall emphasize these differences again later, but for the present we group them together under the label *withdrawals* and use $_nw_x$ as the symbol for the number of cases withdrawn alive (necessarily or otherwise) between time x and time $x + n$. We now examine how cases withdrawn from a study *at the beginning of each interval* affect our original data. For this illustration we also assume that those withdrawn experience the same probability of death after withdrawal as those remaining under observation. These assumptions are reflected in Table 7-3. A column is also provided for a new cumulative survival function, "probability of surviving from time 0 to time $x + 2$."

Note that in Table 7-3 the number of deaths observed in each interval has been reduced in keeping with the assumption that those withdrawn have the same probability of death after withdrawal as those remaining under observation. Thus, in the period beginning at $x = 0$ and having a probability of death during the interval of about $2/3$, we presume that four of the six withdrawals died following withdrawal and subtract these four deaths from the 195 reported in Table 7-1 as the total deaths for this interval. Among those kept under observation, 191 deaths were observed. An additional four deaths occurred among the six withdrawals, and these were not observed. Combining observed and unobserved deaths, we have the same total (195) as in Table 7-1. The column for cumulative probability of survival relates to survival from time 0 to time $x + 2$. Thus, if 12-month survival is desired, the product $\prod_{i=0}^{x/2} {_2p_{2i}}$ uses $x = 10$.

The index then relates to $i = 0,1,2, \ldots, 10/2$, with corresponding values of $_2p_{2i}$ of $_2p_0, _2p_2, _2p_4, \cdots, _2p_{10}$. The calculation for $_2q_x$ in Table 7-3 has been modified to reflect the assumption that the $_nw_x$ are lost to observation at the *beginning of each interval*. Thus, in the first interval, the probability of death is calculated as $191/294$ rather than $191/300$. If $_2w_0$ of the individuals given transplants withdrew from the study immediately following surgery and thus from *any* possibility of being recorded among the $_2d_0$, we calculate the probability of dying among those remaining under observation as

$_2d_0/(O_0 - _2w_0)$. The data presented in Table 7-3 reflect almost (because $_2d_x$ and $_2w_x$ are restricted to integer values) the same probability of dying ($_2q_x$) for those withdrawn as for the total group defined in Table 7-2. In summary, some individuals withdrew alive, but both those who withdrew and those who remained under observation had the same probability of death as experienced by the total group in Table 7-2.

The existence of withdrawals is very much in keeping with real experience and real data. Our stipulation that the withdrawals and those remaining under observation have the same probability of death and that withdrawals all take place exactly at the beginning of an interval are less realistic, but they are included to permit step-by-step explanation of the elements involved in calculating summary statistics.

Note in Table 7-3 that the number observed to be alive at 12 months divided by the number given transplants is $5/300$, or .017, not the .10 that was calculated from Table 7-2 as the probability of survival for the entire group. However, the $_2q_x$ probabilities in Table 7-3 are almost identical with those in Table 7-2. By first calculating $1 - _2q_x = _2p_x$ and then forming the product $_{12}P_0 = \prod_{i=0}^{5} {_2p_{2i}}$, we arrive at .10 as the probability of surviving from surgery to the first anniversary, exactly as in Table 7-2. In this illustration, which includes some withdrawals, it is clear that the product of survival probabilities for individual intervals provides a good estimate of overall survival whereas the number observed to have survived divided by the number given transplants does not. Studies without withdrawals, while deserving of high praise, are extremely rare, and so we concentrate only on the use of the product of interval probabilities of survival to estimate overall survival.

The calculation of each interval probability of death is affected by assumptions regarding withdrawals. Suppose we consider data relating to a one-year interval x to $x + 1$ as O_x, $_1d_x$, and $_1w_x$, with $O_x - _1w_x - _1d_x = O_{x+1}$. When $n = 1$, it is customary to omit it from the notation used, and we shall adopt this convention. Possible assumptions about the w_x individuals are

1. All have died by time $x + 1$
2. None have died by time $x + 1$
3. They experience the same probability of death after withdrawal as those who remain under observation

The first two assumptions tend to be unrealistic, but they permit calculation of limits within which the truth lies. The calculation of q_x under the assumption that all withdrawals died before the end of the interval in which they withdrew (assumption 1) is

$$q_x = \frac{d_x + w_x}{O_x}$$

Table 7-3. Data from Table 7-1 in Life Table Format Modified for Withdrawals at Beginning of Interval

Time at beginning of interval	Under observation at exact time x	Number of deaths observed between x and $x+2$	Number withdrawn between x and $x+2$	Adjusted O_x $(O_x - {_2w_x})$	Probability of Dying during interval $({_2d_x}/O'_x)$	Surviving through interval $(1 - {_2q_x})$	Surviving from time 0 to time $x+2$ $\left(\prod_{i=0}^{x/2} {_2p_{2i}}\right)$
x	O_x	$_2d_x$	$_2w_x$	O'_x	$_2q_x$	$_2p_x$	$_{x+2}p_0$
0	300	19†	6	294	.65	.35	.35
2	103	25	8	95	.26	.74	.26
4	70	11	10	60	.18	.82	.21
6	49	7	10	39	.18	.82	.17
8	31	4	10	21	.19	.81	.14
10	17	2	10	7	.29	.71	.10
12	5						

Under the assumption that none died before the end of the interval in which they withdrew (assumption 2), it is

$$q_x = \frac{d_x}{O_x}$$

Assumption 3 is commonly adopted but much less commonly justified by evidence. If all withdrawals are due to the termination of the observation period and if no change in patient selection or treatment occurs over the study period, assumption 3 is probably justified. In most studies, however, we really do not know how withdrawals differ from those remaining under observation, and the very best studies exert considerable effort to keep withdrawals to a minimum.

We now investigate the effect of assumption 3 on the calculation of q_x. Consider a single individual, included among the w_x, who moved from the area and was thus lost to observation at time $x + 3/4$. If this individual had died at time $x + \frac{1}{4}$ or $x + \frac{1}{2}$, she or he would have been recorded among the d_x. She or he was, in fact, under observation and at risk of being included among the d_x from time x to time $x + \frac{3}{4}$. It is only the time following $x + \frac{3}{4}$ that is lost to observation. If we now shift to consideration of all individuals in w_x and make the assumption that withdrawals occur *uniformly* throughout the interval x to $x + 1$, it follows that, on the average, members of w_x are under observation for half of the interval, and it is necessary to use this fact in calculating q_x.

Under the assumptions that withdrawals are uniformly distributed within the interval with respect to time of withdrawal and that the subsequent experience of withdrawals is the same as those remaining under observation, the applicable formula is

$$q_x = \frac{d_x}{O_x - w_x/2} \qquad (7\text{-}1)$$

This method of calculating q_x removes, from the O_x at risk, only half of the w_x, thus effectively counting half of the w_x as being under observation. Of course, it is not half of the w_x individuals who were at risk of being included among the d_x but rather all of the w_x individuals, each for an average of half an interval.

Equation 7-1 for q_x adjusted for withdrawals can also be derived by estimating the number of deaths among withdrawals and adding this to the observed d_x. Under the assumptions of uniform withdrawal and equal risk for withdrawals and those remaining under observation, the number of deaths occurring among the w_x would be $(w_x/2)q_x$. Risk in the entire O_x group can then be estimated by combining deaths among the w_x with the d_x actually observed. Under the assumptions of uniform withdrawal and equal risk, the number of deaths occurring in the w_x is

$$\frac{w_x}{2}\left(\frac{d_x}{O_x - w_x/2}\right)$$

and our alternative estimate of risk is

$$q'_x = \frac{d_x + \dfrac{w_x}{2}\left(\dfrac{d_x}{O_x - w_x/2}\right)}{O_x} \qquad (7\text{-}2)$$

By multiplying the first term in the numerator by

$$\frac{O_x - \dfrac{w_x}{2}}{O_x - \dfrac{w_x}{2}}$$

q'_x in Equation 7-2 can be shown to be identical to q_x in Equation 7-1:

$$q'_x = \frac{\dfrac{d_x(O_x - w_x/2)}{O_x - w_x/2} + \dfrac{d_x}{O_x - w_x/2}\left(\dfrac{w_x}{2}\right)}{O_x} = \frac{d_xO_x - \dfrac{d_xw_x}{2} + \dfrac{d_xw_x}{2}}{\left(O_x - \dfrac{w_x}{2}\right)O_x}$$

$$= \frac{d_xO_x}{(O_x - \dfrac{w_x}{2})O_x} = \frac{d_x}{O_x - \dfrac{w_x}{2}} = q_x$$

Both equations assume equal probability of death for those withdrawn and those still under observation. Thus

$$q_x = \frac{d_x}{O_x - \dfrac{w_x}{2}}$$

is the probability of death during the interval x to $x + 1$ for those withdrawn, for those remaining under observation, and, consequently, for the total group alive and under observation at the beginning of the interval.

Whenever there is reason to believe that the stipulated assumptions do not apply, the adjustments for withdrawals given in Equations 7-1 and 7-2 are not to be used. The extreme assumptions of all w_x dying or none dying are always possible, although not too often helpful. If you have specific data about time of withdrawals or risk after withdrawal, substitute such data for the "standard" assumptions.

We now repeat the data of Table 7-3 with q_x calculated according to the standard assumptions. This is shown in Table 7-4. As in prior modifications, the original data presented in Table 7-1 have been adjusted in Table 7-4 to fit the assumptions used. For example, in Table 7-4 the six withdrawals in the first interval are now presumed to have been under observation for half the interval.

Thus the approximately $\frac{2}{3}$ probability of death reported for this interval in Table 7-1 results in (6) $(\frac{1}{2})$ $(\frac{2}{3})$ = 2 deaths among the $_2w_0$. The total of 195 deaths reported for $_2d_0$ in Table 7-1 has accordingly been reduced to 193 in Table 7-4.

Although different methods of calculating $_2q_x$ are used in Tables 7-3 and 7-4, each method is in keeping with the assumptions relating to it. The overall results, to two digits, of .10 survival for one year in Table 7-3 and .09 in Table 7-4 differ because of the need to keep to integer values for the number of deaths and not because of any fundamental discrepancy. Withdrawals occurring immediately at the beginning of each interval, as in Table 7-3, are unlikely in real data. They are used solely to introduce the subject of adjustment for withdrawals.

Our discussion on adjustment for withdrawals has been based on two unstated assumptions, which we now specify. The first is that the risk of death is fairly constant within the interval of analysis. For many investigations, this will be the case; in others, it may be possible to approximate this requirement by shortening the interval being analyzed. Note that the approximate constancy of risk within an interval is of concern only when adjustment is required for withdrawals. If no cases are withdrawn, the intervals of analysis can be of any length and there is no requirement of constant risk within them. If there are withdrawals, however, we need a basis for assuming that someone withdrawn for the last $1/k$ of the interval and subject to the same risk as those remaining under observation has $1/k$ the probability of an event applicable to an individual observed over the entire interval. Without this assumption, the use of Equations 7-1 and 7-2 is not justified. Of course, if the nature of the changing risk within the interval is known, alternative estimates of the risk of death among cases withdrawn may be possible. To illustrate the importance of constant risk, consider a life table calculation on survival incorporating birth to age 9.99 years as a single interval. The risk of death during this interval is very heavily concentrated between birth and age one. We further assume a large number of withdrawals exactly at age five; thus the withdrawals were present for the first half of the 0 to 9.99 interval but not for the second half. By using Equations 7-1 and 7-2, we would be incorporating into our estimate of $_{10}q_0$ the idea that the risk during the period lost to observation among the $_{10}w_0$ individuals is proportional to that actually observed over the whole period. This is false, however, and thus Equations 7-1 and 7-2 are not appropriate. This problem can be avoided easily by subdividing the intervals into periods having approximately constant risk.

The second assumption that has been unstated to this point relates to combining data from different calendar periods. For any specific interval of analysis x to $x + n$, if data come from different calendar periods, we must assume that there is no secular trend in risk. The life table method can, and does, distinguish between risks in various time periods following entry. There is no requirement to assume anything as to the nature of risk changes with time after entry. However, if several different calendar periods contribute data on

Table 7-4. Data from Table 7-1 in Life Table Format Modified for Uniform Withdrawals during an Interval

Time at beginning of interval	Under observation at exact time x	Number of deaths observed between x and x+2	Number withdrawn between x and x+2	Adjusted O_x $\left(O_x - \dfrac{_2w_x}{2}\right)$	Probability of		
					Dying during interval $\left(\dfrac{_2d_x}{O'_x}\right)$	Surviving through interval $(1 - {_2q_x})$	Surviving from time 0 to time x+2 $\left(\prod\limits_{i=0}^{x/2} {_2p_{2i}}\right)$
x	O_x	$_2d_x$	$_2w_x$	O'_x	$_2q_x$	$_2p_x$	$_{x+2}P_0$
0	300	193	6	297	.65	.35	.35
2	101	25	8	97	.26	.74	.26
4	68	12	10	63	.19	.81	.21
6	46	8	10	41	.20	.80	.17
8	28	4	10	23	.17	.83	.14
10	14	3	10	9	.33	.67	.09
12	1						

the risk in the *same time interval after entry*, it is necessary to assume that the risk for this interval is not changing over time. If it is, the life table statistics are difficult or impossible to interpret.

In summary, if the study contains cases withdrawn from observation, Equations 7-1 and 7-2 may provide satisfactory estimates if it is reasonable to assume that

1. Those withdrawn do not differ from those continued under observation as to expected mortality both in the interval of withdrawal and in later intervals
2. Within an interval, the risk of death for subintervals of equal length is approximately constant
3. Withdrawals occur uniformly within an interval
4. If data for several different *calendar periods* are being combined into a single interval x to $x + n$, there is no secular trend in risk

We now return to the distinction between withdrawals and losses from observation. Because withdrawals, which occur because of cutoff date for analysis, represent more recent cases, their survival rates may conceivably differ from those of nonwithdrawals, which may represent older patients treated many years ago (see assumption 4 above). However, they are less subject to the myriad biases potentially affecting losses to observation. Although most investigators feel comfortable about the assumption that the future experiences of withdrawals are similar to those of subjects remaining under observation, the only way to feel secure about losses from observation is to have very few of them. The fewer the losses, the less distortion possible in using assumptions that may or may not be justified. If data are available on some characteristics of the lost cases, they can then be compared with cases remaining under observation. Although the prime variable of interest—outcome—remains unknown, comparison of auxiliary variables provides some sense of whether or not lost cases are similar to others. Exactly the same procedure may be followed in comparing withdrawals and cases remaining under observation.

LIFE TABLES FOR SPECIFIC CAUSES

At times the investigator wishes to calculate the probability of death from a particular cause, either with or without adjustment for competing causes. Suppose we are investigating the probability of dying from cancer among those diagnosed as having cancer of a particular type. Persons in the study who are killed in traffic accidents no longer have the possibility of dying from cancer. It is in this sense that the deaths due to traffic and all other noncancer deaths are "competing" with the principal study out-come, i.e., mortality from cancer. We shall call probabilities adjusted for competing causes, net probabilities of death and those not adjusted for competing causes *crude probabilities of death* [75]. We illustrate these calculations by returning to the data of Table 7-4, but with a subdivision of $_2d_x$ data into deaths from heart disease and deaths from all other causes. These subdivided data are shown in Table 7-5. Life table symbols x, O_x, $_nd_x$, $_nw_x$, and $_nq_x$, which have been used several times previously, are used in Table 7-5 without additional labeling. Readers who are doubtful about any of these symbols should refer to Table 7-3.

In Table 7-5 the ratios of heart disease deaths to total deaths for the six intervals beginning with $x = 0$ are .124, .280, .500, .125, .500, and .333. Applying these proportions to the corresponding total $_2q_x$ values results in .081, .072, .095, .024, .087, and .111 as the *crude* probabilities of death from heart disease.

A *net* probability of death from heart disease can be calculated by treating patients who died from all the other causes as if they had been withdrawn alive. By this method, the actual deaths from other causes are "permitted" to die, in the future, of the net cause under the standard assumption that withdrawals are subject to the same risks after withdrawal as those remaining under observation. The assumption that, had they remained alive, patients dying of other causes would have been at no different risk for heart disease than the surviving population is necessary if this procedure is to yield sensible results. Whenever a competing cause is correlated with the net cause—for example, suicide (competing) with cancer mortality (net)—the use of this method becomes questionable. The calculation of net probability of death from heart disease (all other causes not operating) is illustrated in Table 7-6. The net probability of death from heart disease (Table 7-6) is higher in every interval than the crude probability of death from heart disease (Table 7-5). Of course, this is due to the artificial canceling of other causes of death and to the applying of the risk of dying from heart disease both to the living *and* to those dead of other causes.

In his excellent book *Introduction to Stochastic Processes in Bio-statistics* [73], Chiang derives life table functions based on the force of mortality operating over infinitesimal intervals. These same functions are defined herein from the viewpoint of simplicity rather than rigor. We shall use the data reported by Chiang relating to survival following diagnosis of breast cancer to compare calculations described herein with those described by Chiang. These comparisons are shown in Table 7-7. The statistic we use for comparison is the probability of surviving to the tenth anniversary after entry into the study, with respect to three specifically identified risks. The terminology used in this book is slightly different from that used by Chiang, and we report both labelings in Table 7-7.

All calculations of probability of surviving to the tenth anniversary were derived from Chiang's data. The appropriate values of q_x were converted to p_x and then survival to the tenth anniversary was computed as $\prod_{x=0}^{9} p_x$. It is comforting to know that the methods described herein for calculating P_x lead to results that are in substantial agreement with the more precise methods described by Chiang.

Note that for either method of calculation the probability of *surviving* a net risk of death from breast cancer is less than the probability of *surviving* a crude

Table 7-5. Data from Table 7-4 with Subdivision of $_2d_x$ and Calculation of *Crude* Probability for Death from Heart Disease

| | | $_2d_x$ | | | | | $_2q_x$ | |
| | | | | | | | | |
x	O_x	Total	Heart disease	Other	$_2w_x$	O'_x	Total	Heart disease	Other
0	300	193	24	169	6	297	.650	.081	.569
2	101	25	7	18	8	97	.258	.072	.186
4	68	12	6	6	10	63	.190	.095	.095
6	46	8	1	7	10	41	.195	.024	.171
8	28	4	2	2	10	23	.174	.087	.087
10	14	3	1	2	10	9	.333	.111	.222
12	3								

Table 7-6. Data from Table 7-4 with Subdivision of $_2d_x$ and Calculation of *Net* Probability of Death from Heart Disease

x	O_x	$_2d_x$ Heart disease	Other	$_2w_x$	O_x adjusted for net probability from heart disease $\left[O_x - \dfrac{_2w_x}{2} - \dfrac{_2d_x(\text{other})}{2}\right]$ O'_x	Net probability of death from heart disease $[_2d_x(\text{h.d.})/O'_x]$ $_2q_x$ (h.d.)
0	300	24	169	6	212.5	.113
2	101	7	18	8	88.0	.080
4	68	6	6	10	60.0	.100
6	46	1	7	10	37.5	.027
8	28	2	2	10	22.0	.091
10	14	1	2	10	8.0	.125
12	3					

Table 7-7. Computed Probability of Surviving Specific Risks: Comparison of Procedures in This Book with Those of Chiang

Risk	Probability of surviving to tenth anniversary with respect to specified risk	
	Chiang[a]	This book
Net probability of death from breast cancer		.488
Net probability of death from breast cancer acting alone	.486	
Crude probability of death from breast cancer		.493
Partial crude probability of death from breast cancer when risk of being lost is eliminated	.491	
Death from any cause		.363
Net probability of death when risk of being lost is eliminated	.361	

[a] Data from C. L. Chiang, *Introduction to Stochastic Processes in Biostatistics*, p. 292. New York: Wiley, 1968 by permission.

risk of death from breast cancer. This is in agreement with our previous observation that the net probability of *dying* from a specific cause is larger than the crude probability. Note also the very small change from crude to net risk. Unless the competing risks are very large, crude and net risks will be similar.

Kuzma [76] has reported on extensive comparisons of Chiang's method and the Cutler-Ederer method [74], which is equivalent to the life table calculations reported herein. After investigating various rates of withdrawal and various risks of death, Kuzma concluded, "The discrepancy of the two methods was found to be negligible for survival rates and standard errors when the withdrawing rates were $\leqslant 30$ percent and the lost to follow-up rate < 40 percent".

SAMPLING ERROR AND SIGNIFICANCE TESTS

Life table functions, as any other statistics, are subject to sampling error. Consider $_x\hat{P}_0$, the estimated probability of surviving several intervals from time 0 to time x. Had different individuals been included in our sample data, we very likely would have different results. In calculating the standard error of $_x\hat{P}_0$, we are estimating the standard deviation of the distribution of all possible $_x\hat{P}_0$ values resulting from all possible samples of 300 from the universe† of individuals given cardiac transplants. Greenwood's formula for the standard error of $_{x+1}\hat{P}_0$ is [77]

$$\hat{SE}(_{x+1}P_0) = {_{x+1}}\hat{P}_0 \sqrt{\sum_{i=0}^{x} \frac{q_i}{O'_i - d_i}} \qquad (7\text{-}3)$$

As written, Equation 7-3 relates to $_{x+1}\hat{P}_0$ calculated from p_x values for one-year (or one-month) intervals. We can rewrite it to fit the data in Table 7-4 based on two-month intervals:

$$\hat{SE}(_{x+2}P_0) = {}_{x+2}\hat{P}_0 \sqrt{\sum_{i=0}^{x/2} \frac{{}_2 q_{2i}}{O'_{2i} - {}_2 d_{2i}}} \qquad (7\text{-}4)$$

Note that Equation 7-3 pertains to survival from time 0 to time $x+1$ and Equation 7-4 pertains to survival from time 0 to time $x + 2$. Select the value of x appropriate for the period you wish to analyze. Applying Equation 7-4 to the data in Table 7-4, we get

$$\hat{SE}(_2P_0) = .35 \sqrt{\frac{.65}{297 - 193}} = .0277$$

$$\hat{SE}(_4P_0) = .26 \sqrt{\frac{.65}{297 - 193} + \frac{.26}{97 - 25}} = .0258$$

$$\hat{SE}(_6P_0) = .21 \sqrt{\frac{.65}{297 - 193} + \frac{.26}{97 - 25} + \frac{.19}{63 - 12}} = .0245$$

$$\hat{SE}(_8P_0) = .17 \sqrt{\frac{.65}{297 - 193} + \frac{.26}{97 - 25} + \frac{.19}{63 - 12} + \frac{.20}{41 - 8}} = .0238$$

$$\hat{SE}(_{10}P_0) = .14 \sqrt{\frac{.65}{297 - 193} + \frac{.26}{97 - 25} + \frac{.19}{63 - 12} + \frac{.20}{41 - 8} + \frac{.17}{23 - 4}}$$

$$= .0237$$

$$\hat{SE}(_{12}P_0) =$$

$$.09 \sqrt{\frac{.65}{297 - 193} + \frac{.26}{97 - 25} + \frac{.19}{63 - 12} + \frac{.20}{41 - 8} + \frac{.17}{23 - 4} + \frac{.33}{9 - 3}} = .0260$$

When

$$\frac{\hat{SE}(_{x+n}P_0)}{_{x+n}\hat{P}_0}$$

is $\frac{1}{3}$ or less and $_n d_x$ is 10 or greater, the assumption that the sampling distribution of $_{x+n}\hat{P}_0$ is approximately normal is a reasonable one and $\hat{SE}(_{x+n}P_0)$ can be used to establish confidence limits on $_{x+n}P_0$ as was done with $\bar{x}$ in Equations 1-19 and 1-20:

$$_{x+n}\hat{P}_0 \pm 1.96\ \hat{SE}(_{x+n}P_0) = 95\% \text{ CL for } _{x+n}P_0$$

$$_{x+n}\hat{P}_0 \pm 2.58\ \hat{SE}(_{x+n}P_0) = 99\% \text{ CL for } _{x+n}P_0$$

where $_{x+n}P_0$ is the true value for survival from time 0 to time $x + n$ in the universe being sampled. If either or both of the conditions—$\hat{SE}(_{x+n}P_0)/_{x+n}\hat{P}_0$ $\leqslant 1/3$ and $_nd_x \geqslant 10$—are not met, then the assumption as to normality of the sampling distribution cannot be taken for granted.

Standard errors for $_{x+1}P_0$ can be used for establishing confidence limits as described above or can be used to test whether two groups differ significantly in proportion surviving from time 0 to time $x + 1$. The test makes use of Equation 1-9:

$$\text{var}(x - y) = \text{var}(x) + \text{var}(y)$$

if x and y are independent.

For our present interest in comparing $_{x+1}\hat{P}_0$ for groups a and b, which we designate $_{x+1}\hat{P}_{0a}$ and $_{x+1}\hat{P}_{0b}$, respectively, we have

$$\text{var}(_{x+1}P_{0a} - {_{x+1}}P_{0b}) = \text{var}(_{x+1}P_{0a}) + \text{var}(_{x+1}P_{0b})$$

Since $_{x+1}\hat{P}_{0a}$ and $_{x+1}\hat{P}_{0b}$ are derived from different populations, it is reasonable to assume that they are independent variables (e.g., if we know that our sample value of $_{x+1}\hat{P}_{0a}$ happens to be higher than the population parameter it estimates, this knowledge provides no basis for concluding that our sample value of $_{x+1}\hat{P}_{0b}$ is therefore likely to be higher, or lower, than the population parameter it is estimating).

Since the standard error of a statistic is the standard deviation of its sampling distribution (Chapter 1), the variance of that statistic is simply the square of its standard error:

$$\text{var}(_{x+1}P_{0a}) = [\text{SE}(_{x+1}P_{0a})]^2$$

Conversely, the standard error of a statistic is the square root of its variance. Therefore the difference minus the expected value of the difference (equal to zero under the null hypothesis) divided by the square root of the variance of the difference, under the null hypothesis and the usual constraints of adequate sample size, is distributed as a standardized normal deviate and can be tested as such:

$$\frac{(_{x+1}\hat{P}_{0a} - {_{x+1}}\hat{P}_{0b}) - 0}{\{[\hat{SE}(_{x+1}P_{0a})]^2 + [\hat{SE}(_{x+1}P_{0b})]^2\}^{1/2}} = z$$

Before discussing other methods for evaluating whether or not life tables differ significantly, let us outline the general characteristics of these alternative approaches. In contrast to the calculation of standard error for a specific survival time, both the Mantel-Haenszel procedure [47, 78] and the logrank method [78, 79] compare the two survival curves over the entire period being analyzed. For example, consider the two survival curves labeled A and B in

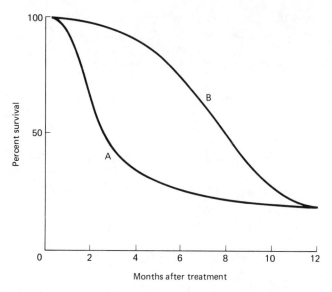

Figure 7-1. Survival curves that differ greatly prior to a point of equality.

Figure 7-1. At the 12-month anniversary, the survival for group A is equal to that for group B, but this equal survival for A has just appeared. At two, four, six, eight, and ten months, B had better survival. Under these conditions, the simple comparison at 12 months misses a great deal of the information that is used by the two alternative methods we now discuss.

The M-H method for obtaining a summary χ^2 from a series of 2 × 2 tables is an excellent method for judging whether two life tables differ by more than can be reasonably attributed to chance. Theoretical justification for treating each life table interval as a separate stratum and comparing the two life tables within each stratum according to the M-H procedure is given by Mantel[78]. For illustration, let us assume that we have life table data on two groups, m and n, as in Table 7-8. For each interval in Table 7-8, a 2 × 2 table can be constructed as

Table 7-8. Comparison of Life Table Data for Groups m and n

x	O'_x (no. at risk) m	O'_x (no. at risk) n	$_2d_x$ (deaths) m	$_2d_x$ (deaths) n	$O'_x - _2d_x$ (survivors) m	$O'_x - _2d_x$ (survivors) n	$_{x+2}P_0$ (probability of surviving to $x + 2$) m	$_{x+2}P_0$ (probability of surviving to $x + 2$) n
0	297	297	193	165	104	132	.350	.444
2	97	132	25	30	72	102	.260	.343
4	63	102	12	15	51	87	.210	.293
6	41	87	8	15	33	72	.169	.242
8	23	72	4	11	19	61	.140	.205
10	9	61	3	17	6	44	.093	.148
Total			245	253				

Table 7-9. Basic Life Table Data Arranged in 2×2 Table Format[a]

Group	Died	Survived	Total at risk
m	193 (a)	104 (b)	297 (m_1)
n	165 (c)	132 (d)	297 (m_2)
Total	358 (n_1)	236 (n_2)	594 (t)

[a] Data are from Table 7-8 for the interval beginning at time $x = 0$.

shown in Table 7-9 for the interval beginning at $x = 0$. For each cell and marginal total in Table 7-9, there is shown in parentheses the notation used extensively in Chapter 5 on adjustment of data. The odds ratio calculation, as in the more general examples discussed earlier, is

$$\hat{OR} = \frac{\sum_i a_i d_i / t_i}{\sum_i b_i c_i / t_i}$$

In this case $\hat{OR}$ refers to the odds of dying for those in group m compared with those in group n. The summations extend over all intervals to be included in the comparison. This is usually the full set of data, but it is possible to compare life tables for only part of the full period (e.g., from $x = 2$ to $x = 6$).

The overall significance test comparing group m with group n with respect to risk of death is based on

$$\chi^2_{1df} = \frac{[|\sum a_i - \sum (Ea_i)| - \frac{1}{2}]^2}{\sum \text{var}(a_i)}$$

as explained and illustrated in Chapter 5. Using Table 7-8 data to compute the overall odds ratio and the overall χ^2_{1df} according to the M-H procedure, we get

$$\hat{OR} = 1.37$$

$$\chi^2_1 = 5.66$$

Thus, group m is estimated to be about 1.4 times as risky as group n with respect to the odds of dying. Furthermore this estimated odds ratio is unlikely to result simply by chance because the probability of a χ^2 with one degree of freedom being as large as or larger than 5.66 when the null hypothesis of no difference between groups is true is less than .02.

Recalling that the M-H odds ratio estimates (a) the common odds ratio if there is one or (b) a reasonably weighted average of the separate odds ratios in the different strata otherwise, this method, like all epidemiologic methods, needs to be applied with understanding. If the two survival curves have, as in

Figure 7-1, no crossover or at most trivival amount of crossover, comparison according to the M-H summary chi square can be useful. But what of survival curves that cross over to the extent that, during the first half of the study, results are exactly the opposite of those during the second half? In this situation an M-H summary indicating little difference overall is obviously misleading. Averages are most useful and informative when derived from similar quantities, and like all other averages the M-H summary can be misleading if used thoughtlessly.

Another method for an overall statistical comparison of life tables is the logrank test. This was first reported by Mantel as a rank order statistic dependent only on the ranking of time of death of individuals in the two groups [78]. The name *logrank* and details of the computation of approximate χ^2 values for this test come from Peto et al. [79]. Although it is presented as a test arising from small intervals of analysis (such as single days or periods encompassing only one death), it is suitable for analyzing data in more common and somewhat longer intervals, provided that the proportion dying within any interval is small (less than 10 percent).

We shall describe the logrank method, illustrate its application to ordinary interval summary data, and then compare the logrank approximate χ^2 values with M-H χ^2 values. In order to demonstrate the conditions under which these two χ^2 values are very similar, we compare intervals in which the risk is high with intervals without high levels of risk.

As described by Peto et al. [79], the logrank method depends on the number at risk at the beginning of each interval. Thus, using Table 7-8 notation, O'_{xm} and O'_{xn} are at risk for the period beginning at time x in groups m and n respectively. The expected number of deaths in each interval for each group is equal to the same proportion of the total deaths $(d_{xm} + d_{xn})$ as each group's proportion of the total number at risk $(O'_{xm} + O'_{xn})$. Therefore the expected number of deaths in group m for the period beginning at time x is

$$E(d_{xm}) = \frac{O'_{xm}}{O'_{xm} + O'_{xn}} (d_{xm} + d_{xn})$$

Similarly,

$$E(d_{xn}) = \frac{O'_{xn}}{O'_{xm} + O'_{xn}} (d_{xm} + d_{xn})$$

Under the null hypothesis of no difference in survival between groups m and n, the expectation that the group with the larger number of individuals at risk at the beginning of an interval will have the larger number of deaths in that interval is both simple and intuitively appealing. By this process, the expected number of deaths is derived for each interval of each life table. It is then an easy matter to compare the *total observed* number of deaths from each life table with the *total expected* number of deaths for the same life table. Totals are obtained from all intervals to be included in the analysis.

Under the null hypothesis (and the assumption of very small intervals of analysis or low interval risk), the square of the difference between total observed deaths and total expected deaths divided by the total expected deaths summed for two groups is approximately χ^2 with one degree of freedom. For groups m and n, this is

$$\chi_1^2 \cong \frac{\left[\sum_x d_{xm} - \sum_x E(d_{xm})\right]^2}{\sum_x E(d_{xm})} + \frac{\left[\sum_x d_{xn} - \sum_x E(d_{xn})\right]^2}{\sum_x E(d_{xn})}$$

In general, if k life tables are being compared to see if they differ by more than can be readily attributed to chance, we can compute

$$\chi_{k-1}^2 \cong \sum_{i=1}^{k} \frac{\left(\begin{array}{c}\text{total observed} \\ \text{deaths in } i\end{array} - \begin{array}{c}\text{total expected} \\ \text{deaths in } i\end{array}\right)^2}{\text{total expected deaths in } i} \tag{7-5}$$

where i represents the ith life table and *total* refers to the total over the life table intervals being evaluated. Within each interval the expected number of deaths in group i is obtained by multiplying the total number of deaths $d_{x\,(\text{total})}$ by the ratio $O'_{xi}/O'_{x\,(\text{total})}$. The statistical significance of life table comparisons is then evaluated by referring to a table of chi square values to determine if the χ^2 calculated is or is not unusual (for the appropriate number of degrees of freedom).

A numeric illustration will clarify how the logrank method is used. To this end we compare life table data for two groups. In Table 7-10, columns 1 and 2 are taken from basic life table data for two groups, r and s. Column 3 expresses how the total at risk within each interval is proportionately distributed between groups r and s. Expected numbers of deaths are derived by multiplying the *total* number of deaths in column 2 by the proportionate distribution of the total number at risk in column 3. Thus, for the interval beginning at time 0, the expected number of deaths in group r is $45(.667) = 30.02$ and in group s is $45(.333) = 14.98$. To compare the two groups over the period from time 0 to time 6 requires summation of all deaths and expected deaths over this interval. These sums are shown in Table 7-10 on the "total" line. Note that deaths or expected deaths in the interval *beginning* at time 6 do not belong in the above comparison and are properly omitted. Using Table 7-10 data for this specific comparison of groups r and s, we get

$$\chi_1^2 \cong \frac{(36 - 42.95)^2}{42.95} + \frac{(28 - 21.05)^2}{21.05} \cong 3.42$$

Table 7-10. Basic Life Table Data and Work Sheet for Logrank Comparison of Groups r and s

| | (1) | | | (2) | | | (3) | | (2 total) × (3) | |
| | O'_x (no. at risk) | | | d_x (deaths) | | | Proportion of O'_x total in | | Expected deaths under null hypothesis | |
x	r	s	Total	r	s	Total	r	s	r	s
0	300	150	450	25	20	45	.667	.333	30.02	14.98
1	275	130	405	4	3	7	.679	.321	4.75	2.25
2	271	127	398	3	2	5	.681	.319	3.40	1.60
3	268	125	393	1	1	2	.682	.318	1.36	.64
4	267	124	391	2	1	3	.683	.317	2.05	.95
5	265	123	388	1	1	2	.683	.317	1.37	.63
6	264	122	386	—	—	—	—	—	—	—
Total				36	28	64			42.95	21.05

To compare two life tables, the formal equation in accordance with Equation 7-5 with $k = 2$ is

$$\chi_1^2 \cong \sum_{i=1}^{2} \frac{\left[\sum_{j=1}^{t} O_{ij} - \sum_{j=1}^{t} E(d_{ij}) \right]^2}{\sum_{j=1}^{t} E(d_{ij})} \tag{7-6}$$

where

$$i = 1, 2 = \text{groups being compared}$$
$$j = 1, 2, \ldots, t = \text{life table intervals being evaluated}$$
$$O_{ij} = \text{observed deaths in } j\text{th interval of } i\text{th group}$$
$$E(d_{ij}) = \text{expected deaths in } j\text{th interval of } i\text{th group}$$

The logrank method (and the M-H method as well) can be used to compare survival curves over any interval of interest. All that is necessary is to set the index of summation to fit the interval to be evaluated:

$$\sum_{j=0}^{x}, \sum_{j=x}^{x+\Delta}, \text{etc.}$$

The logrank method is excellent, and an approximate summary χ^2 derived from it is easy to calculate, but this method can be misleading if the need to avoid intervals of high risk is forgotten. To demonstrate this, we shall compare summary χ^2 values obtained from logrank and from M-H procedures for different sets of data. We begin by considering the data in Table 7-8, which clearly violate the logrank requirement for low-risk intervals (e.g., in the interval beginning at time $x = 0$, $_2q_{0(m)} = 193/297 = .65$ and $_2q_{0(n)} = 165/297 = .56$. Table 7-11 presents the data from Table 7-8 in a form convenient for logrank calculations. Using Equation 7-5 and the total observed and total expected deaths in Table 7-11, we get a one-degree-of-freedom, approximate summary χ^2 comparing groups m and n by logrank methods:

$$\chi_1^2 \text{ (logrank)} \cong \frac{(245 - 226.20)^2}{226.20} + \frac{(253 - 271.80)^2}{271.80} = 2.86$$

We previously calculated a M-H χ^2 using the same data to compare groups m and n and found χ_1^2 (M-H) = 5.66. This discrepancy for χ^2 is substantial and can be attributed to an inappropriate use of the logrank method.

We now compare iogrank and M-H calculations of summary χ^2 values using Table 7-10 data. For this purpose we show Table 7-12 with data derived from Table 7-10 and labeled to show cells a_i, b_i, c_i, d_i, etc., as follows:

	Deaths	Survivors	At risk
Group r	a_i	b_i	m_{1i}
Group s	c_i	d_i	m_{2i}
Total	n_{1i}	n_{2i}	t_i

Using Table 7-12 data and the M-H procedure, we get $\chi_1^2 = 3.16$. This is quite similar to the χ_1^2 value of 3.42 obtained with the logrank procedure on these same data. In fact, the values are so close that their relationship (i.e., which

Table 7-11. Basic Life Table Data from Table 7-8 and Work Sheet for Logrank Comparison of Groups m and n

	(1)			(2)			(3) Proportion of O'_x total in		(4) Expected deaths under null hypothesis	
	O'_x (no. at risk)			$_2d_x$ (deaths)						
x	m	n	Total	m	n	Total	m	n	m	n
0	297	297	594	193	165	358	.500	.500	179.00	179.00
2	97	132	229	25	30	55	.424	.576	23.32	31.68
4	63	102	165	12	15	27	.382	.618	10.31	16.69
6	41	87	128	8	15	23	.320	.680	7.36	15.64
8	23	72	95	4	11	15	.242	.758	3.63	11.37
10	9	61	70	3	17	20	.129	.871	2.58	17.42
Total	—	—	—	245	253	498	—	—	226.20	271.80

Table 7-12. Basic Life Table Data from Table 7-10 Arranged for Mantel-Haenszel Computations

	Group "r"			Group "s"			Total		
i	Deaths (a_i)	Survivors (b_i)	At risk (m_{1i})	Deaths (c_i)	Survivors (d_i)	At risk (m_{2i})	Deaths (n_{1i})	Survivors (n_{2i})	At risk (t_i)
0	25	275	300	20	130	150	45	405	450
1	4	271	275	3	127	130	7	398	405
2	3	268	271	2	125	127	5	393	398
3	1	267	268	1	124	125	2	391	393
4	2	265	267	1	123	124	3	388	391
5	1	264	265	1	122	123	2	386	388

of the two is larger) is determined by the use or avoidance of the $\frac{1}{2}$ "continuity correction" used in the M-H calculation but not in the logrank method. Thus, in this instance, with no $_2q_x$ value greater than .133 (20/150 for group s in the period beginning at time $x = 0$) and most considerably lower, the logrank χ^2 computation is entirely satisfactory.

DEMOGRAPHIC LIFE TABLES

There are two major types of life tables: one is called medical, clinical, or cohort and the other demographic. All the description and discussion of life tables to this point relates to medical life tables derived from data on a real cohort. The demographic life table, computed on the basis of national (or regional) mortality data, is obtained by *applying the currently observed mortality risks at various ages to an imaginary cohort.* Thus the expectation of life at birth in the United States, which was 73.3 for 1978 [80], depends on the assumption that a group born in 1978 will be exposed to 1978 age-specific risks of mortality as they go through life (e.g., when this group is age 30 in the year 2008, they will experience the 1978 mortality risks for 30 years olds). Although taken literally this presumption is unrealistic, the demographic life table is an excellent way of summarizing current mortality risks. While epidemiologists in certain specialized areas may use demographic life tables extensively, the medical life table is the one that is more likely to be prepared and analyzed by most epidemiologists. The two types are essentially similar in concept, with national or regional demographic life tables almost always prepared by governmental statistical bureaus. The literature on demographic life tables is enormous and can be complicated. A good general reference is Shryock and Siegel [81].

NOTES

* The joint probability of surviving consecutive intervals uses the basic probability formula $P(AB) = P(A)P(B/A)$, where $P(A)$ represents the probability of surviving the first period,

$P(B/A)$ represents the probability of surviving the second period *given* that the first was survived, and $P(AB)$ represents the probability of surviving both periods. If withdrawals do not complicate the calculation, this relationship can be illustrated with a simple example. If 100 are observed at time 0 and 80 of these survive to time 1, $P(A) = 80/100$. If, *of the 80 surviving to time 1*, 40 survive to time 2, $P(B/A) = 40/80$. The probability of surviving both periods is then the product: $80/100(40/80) = 40/100$. Since all the $_np_x$ values are conditional probabilities, the same calculations and logic apply to a chain of three or more intervals.

† Often the "universe" is poorly described or not described at all, leaving it unclear as to whether the sample at hand is a sample in time, in space, or of surgeons. All extrapolations from the universe sampled to other universes of interest are matters of scientific judgment and are not based on statistical considerations.

8

Longitudinal Studies: Person-Years

The life table method permits us to combine data on those observed for any length of time with data on those observed for longer or shorter periods. Such data can also be combined using the person-years method. I shall first describe this method and then indicate similarities and differences between it and the life table method and suggest how to choose between them.

COMPUTATIONS AND ASSUMPTIONS

Suppose we wish to estimate the annual incidence rate for disabling cataract and have observed two groups. In the first group, observed for one year, the number of persons varies from month to month but averages 500 persons at risk, with 13 developing cataract. In the second group, observed for two years, the size of the group averages 400 persons at risk, with 23 developing cataract. Although the average number of individuals at risk is 900, the number of person-years observed is 500 + 800 = 1300. In order to combine the cataract incidence data from the two groups in a sensible way, two conditions must apply:

1. Risk must increase proportionately as length of observation increases.
2. Individuals in each group must be at similar risk.

These conditions are met in some studies, but if it is not reasonable to assume that they are, then the person-years method cannot be used.

If cataract incidence is about 3 percent per year for persons at risk (those without cataract) at about age 70 and if all 900 individuals are age 69 to 71, then both conditions 1 and 2 are met and the person-year method is appropriate. If the individuals are all age 69 to 71 but one-year cataract incidence at age 70 is 60 percent of those at risk instead of 3 percent, person-years would not be appropriate because, at 60 percent risk for a single year, the two-year risk could obviously not be double that for one year. If the 500 individuals observed for one year are age 70 and the 400 observed for two years are age 17, again the person-year method would be inapplicable as cataract risk is known to increase with age. Thus the two groups would not have a similar risk. In order to *pool* observations of different groups for varying periods of time, both conditions listed above must be satisfied.

In our cataract example, the incidence rate of disabling cataract per person-year at risk can be estimated as

$$\frac{13 + 23}{500 + 800} = \frac{36}{1300} = .028 \text{ per person-year at risk}$$

Note that this is an incidence *rate* of acquiring cataract, not a probability. The distinction is simple. A probability, $q_x = d_x/O_x$, relates a number of events during an interval to the number *at risk at the beginning* of the interval. A rate, $m_x = d_x/P_x$, where P_x equals the *average population at risk* during the interval, is based on a different denominator. If the event being counted is death, the probability of death and the rate of death are usually unequal (the rate being greater) because the number under observation at the start of an interval (O_x) is reduced by deaths during the interval. This makes the average number under observation during the period, P_x, less than O_x.*

Similarly, for an event like disabling cataract in either eye, the number under observation and at risk at the start of an interval is reduced during the interval by those developing cataract because these people are no longer at risk of becoming an incident case. For identical starting populations, the rate of a specified event is always larger than (or equal to) the probability of the same event. If we assume that the events are uniformly distributed during the interval, the relationship between q_x (probability) and m_x (rate) can be understood from the following two equations:

$$m_x = q_x \left(\frac{O_x}{O_x - \dfrac{d_x}{2}} \right) \tag{8-1}$$

$$q_x = m_x \left(\frac{PY}{PY + \dfrac{d_x}{2}} \right) \tag{8-2}$$

where *PY* is person-years under observation. The factor

$$\frac{O_x}{O_x - \dfrac{d_x}{2}}$$

is always $\geqslant 1$ and the factor

$$\frac{PY}{PY + \dfrac{d_x}{2}}$$

is always $\leqslant 1$, but since in most practical examples both are very close to unity, the numeric difference between q_x and m_x is usually slight. Only in the case of events having very high risk (i.e., $d_x/2$ equals an appreciable fraction of O_x) do q_x and m_x differ to any practical extent. To illustrate, if the annual probability of death at age 70 is about .05 and at 80 about .12 and assuming uniform distribution of deaths during the year (possibly a questionable assumption at age 80), then

$$m_{70} = .05\left(\frac{100}{100 - 2.5}\right) = .051 \qquad \text{(compared to .050 for } q_{70}\text{)}$$

$$m_{80} = .12\left(\frac{100}{100 - 6}\right) = .128 \qquad \text{(compared to .120 for } q_{80}\text{)}$$

Thus even for the high mortality risk associated with age 80 the distinction between rate and probability is not very great. The direct relationship between q_x and m_x (under the assumption of uniform distribution of events and no withdrawals during the interval x to $x + 1$) is derived as follows. First, we know that

$$q_x = \frac{d_x}{O_x}$$

Since the midpoint between O_x and O_{x+1} is the average population size, $O_x - (d_x/2)$, which we denote by P_x, we can write

$$q_x = \frac{d_x}{P_x + \dfrac{d_x}{2}} = \frac{d_x/P_x}{P_x/P_x + \dfrac{d_x/P_x}{2}}$$

$$= \frac{m_x}{1 + \dfrac{m_x}{2}} = \frac{2m_x}{2 + m_x} \qquad (8\text{-}3)$$

The conditions stated above for using the person-years method made no reference to withdrawals, i.e., persons lost from observation before occurrence of the event being studied. As discussed in Chapter 7 on life tables, these are of two kinds: (a) withdrawals from observation because the cutoff date for analysis is reached and (b) withdrawals from observation because the individual has moved from the study area or cannot be located or does not cooperate as required.

If there are withdrawals, the assumptions required for person-year calculations are the same as for the life table method. These are (a) withdrawals occur uniformly throughout the interval of analysis (so that simple estimates of average population at risk are possible) and (b) the experience of persons after withdrawal is the same as that of persons remaining under observation. As in the case of life table analysis, it is probably more correct to assume equivalent future experience for withdrawals due to cutoff date than for withdrawals lost to observation.

Two other assumptions required for life table calculations are also needed for person-year tabulations. Whether or not there are withdrawals, person-year tabulations require approximate uniformity of risk within the intervals in which data are summarized. The final assumption required for both life table and person-year analyses is that there be no secular trend in data pooled into a common interval.

A practical consequence of the assumption that, within intervals of analysis, the risk is directly proportional to the length of the interval is the need to avoid long intervals. Thus, if we consider the risk of lung cancer among cigarette smokers age 45 to 64, it is unreasonable to suppose that individuals observed for 20 years from age 45 to 64 are subject to only 20 times as much risk from lung cancer as individuals observed for one year beginning at age 45. Pooling such disparate risks into a person-year summary is likely to result in more confusion than enlightenment. If instead of using a 20-year interval, these data were summarized into 5-year intervals (45 to 49, 50 to 54, 55 to 59, and 60 to 64), the combining of person-years observation at the young end of the 5-year interval with observation over the entire 5-year interval or even only with observation at the old end of the 5-year interval may not seriously contradict the requirement that, within intervals, risk be directly proportional to length of observation.

It is essential not to confuse the requirement for constant risk *within an interval* with the requirement for constant risk over the entire age range under study. For example, we may have observation on one individual from age 40 to 54 and on another from age 50 to 59. If the risks within the five-year intervals are approximately constant, pooling within these five-year periods is satisfactory. There is no requirement that risk be constant from age 40 to 59. It is only *within* intervals of analysis that pooling of person-year observation periods takes place, and thus it is only *within* intervals of analysis that the condition of constant risk applies. If there is constant risk within a short or moderately long interval of analysis, then the risk within any subinterval will be closely proportional to the length of observation.

The typical study for which person-year analysis is appropriate concerns a group coming under observation at different ages and remaining under observation for varying periods of time. We first present detailed methods for calculating person-years of observation for age-specific periods, 35 to 44, 45 to 54, etc. This is useful for understanding the procedure and can also be the approach used if computer assistance is available. For illustrative purposes, we shall calculate age-specific risks of lung cancer mortality among six individuals who are regular cigarette smokers. The basic data are shown in Table 8-1. The first step is to convert date on which observation began to age at which

Table 8-1. Data for Calculation of Person-Years of Observation for Six Individuals

Individual	Date of birth	Date observation began	Date observation ended	Lung cancer mortality (0 = no, 1 = yes)
1	Jan. 4, 1897	July 11, 1954	Dec. 31, 1962	0
2	Sept. 5, 1884	Aug. 3, 1954	Nov. 25, 1960	1
3	Dec. 16, 1904	Oct. 25, 1954	Dec. 31, 1962	0
4	Jan. 16, 1899	Nov. 1, 1954	Dec. 31, 1962	0
5	Apr. 9, 1912	Feb. 19, 1957	Dec. 31, 1962	0
6	Feb. 22, 1910	Dec. 8, 1957	Aug. 18, 1959	1

observation began. We do this by subtracting date of birth from date
observation began:

1. Subtraction when no "borrowing" required

Year	Month	Day	
1954	7	11	Date observation began
1897	1	4	Date of birth
57	6	7	Age observation began

2. Subtraction with "borrowing"

Year	Month	Day	
1954	8	3	Date observation began in original units
1953	19	33	Date observation began after subtraction of 1 year and addition of 11 months and 30 days
1884	9	5	Date of birth
69	10	28	Age observation began

By a similar process of subtracting date of birth from date on which
observation terminated, we obtain the individual's age at the time observation
terminated. Table 8-2 presents both beginning and terminating ages for all six
individuals. Also in Table 8-2 are the lengths of observation periods allocated
to the age-specific intervals for which data are being pooled. These are obtained
by defining the beginning and ending ages of the intervals as 45 years, 0 months,
0 days and 54 years, 11 months, 30 days for age 45 to 54; 55 years, 0 months, 0
days and 64 years, 11 months, 30 days for age 55 to 64; and 65 years, 0 months, 0
days and 74 years, 11 months, 30 days for age 65 to 74 and subtracting as
appropriate. The beginning date of observation for individual 1 completely
avoids the 45 to 54 interval, but in the 55 to 64 interval we have

Year	Month	Day	
64	11	30	Ending age observed in interval
57	6	7	Beginning age observed in interval
7	5	23	Time in 55 to 64 interval for individual 1

and in the 65 to 74 interval we have

Year	Month	Day	
65	11	27	Ending age observed in interval
65	0	0	Beginning age observed in interval
0	11	27	Time in 65 to 74 interval for individual 1

Table 8-2. Conversion of Age Observation Began and Age Observation Terminated to Age-Specific Observation Periods

Individual	Age when observation						Length of observation at age								
	Began			Terminated			45–54			55–64			65–74		
	Yr	Mo	Day	Yr	Mo	Day	Yr	Mo	Day	Yr	Mo	Day	Yr	Mo	Day
1	57	6	7	65	11	27	—	—	—	7	5	23	0	11	27
2	69	10	28	76	2	20	—	—	—	—	—	—	5	1	2
3	49	10	9	58	0	15	5	1	21	3	0	15	—	—	—
4	55	9	15	63	11	15	—	—	—	8	2	0	—	—	—
5	44	10	10	50	8	22	5	8	22	—	—	—	—	—	—
6	47	9	16	49	5	26	1	8	10	—	—	—	—	—	—
Total							11	17	53	18	7	38	5	12	29
Person-years[a]								12.56			18.69			6.08	

[a] One month = .08333 years; one day = .00274 years.

Note that, in the 55 to 64 interval, individual 1 is observed until the terminal age for that interval. In the 65 to 74 interval, individual 1 is observed not to the ending age of the interval but to the terminal age of his or her observation in the study. The calculation of length of observation for each of the other five individuals is carried out in a similar way. The rather obvious rules for calculating the length of observation in terms of each age-specific period are

1. For observation beginning within an interval and extending beyond it, subtract the beginning age of observation from the interval ending age.
2. For observation beginning at the start of an interval and ending within it, subtract the beginning age of the interval from the age at which observation is ended.
3. For observation beginning and ending within an interval, subtract the beginning age of observation from the ending age of observation.
4. For observation beginning at the start and continuing to the end of an interval, use the length of the interval.

Summing the years, months, and days contributed by each individual and then converting months and days to person-years, we obtain the total person-years of observation in each ten-year age class, as shown on the bottom line of Table 8.2.

While this detailed approach to calculating person-years of observation for each age class is always possible, and with the aid of computer processing is not unduly difficult, it is not always necessary. Various approximations and simplifications are possible. If the data set is not too large, the hand tally method illustrated in Table 8-3 is commonly used to summarize the age data given in Table 8-2. In Table 8-3, five-year age groupings for year observation began are cross-classified with five-year age groupings for year observation ended, with the number of individuals so classified tallied in each cell. If observation terminated because of death, the tally is in brackets. In the extreme right column of Table 8.3 are the total number of individuals whose observation started during the five-year periods beginning with x as specified. Thus, observation started on one individual during the five-year period beginning with $x = 40$ and on two individuals during the five-year period beginning with $x = 45$. In the bottom two rows are the cases withdrawn alive during each five-year period ($_5w_x$) and the cases dying during each five-year period ($_5d_x$). Those cells for which the age class for beginning observation is identical to the age class for ending observation are shaded for easy identification and later use. Approximate person-years of observation from x to $x + n$ are defined according to Equation 8-4:

$$_nL_x = nO_x + \tfrac{n}{2}\left(_na_x - _nw_x - _nd_x\right) + \tfrac{n}{4}\left(_naw_x + _nad_x\right) \qquad (8\text{-}4)$$

Table 8-3. Work Sheet for Summarizing Person-Year Data

Observation started during 5-year period beginning with x equal to	Observation ended during 5-year period beginning with x equal to								Additions[a] $(_5a_x)$
	40	45	50	55	60	65	70	75	
40			1						1
45		[1]		1					2
50									0
55					1				2
60						1			0
65								[1]	1
70									0
75									0
$_5w_x$	0	0	1	1	1	1	0	0	
$_5d_x$	0	1	0	0	0	0	0	1	

[a] Total number of individuals whose observation started during interval.

where

$_nL_x$ = approximate person-years of observation from age x to age $x + n$

n = length of interval under consideration

O_x = number of individuals under observation at exact age x

$_na_x$ = number of individuals added to those under observation in the age interval x to $x + n$; includes all such individuals whether or not withdrawn or died in the same age interval as added to observation

$_nw_x$ = number of individuals withdrawn alive (whether due to study cutoff date or to loss from observation) during age interval x to $x + n$; includes all such individuals whether or not added to observation in the same age interval as withdrawn

$_nd_x$ = number of deaths during age interval x to $x + n$; includes all such individuals, whether or not they died in the same age interval as added to observation

$_naw_x$ = number of individuals added and withdrawn in the same time interval

$_nad_x$ = number of individuals added and died in the same time interval

I shall first explain Equation 8-4 and then illustrate how the summary columns and rows of Table 8-3 provide the data required by the formula.

Equation 8-4 totals the person-years of observation from x to $x + n$ as follows. The first term, nO_x, counts n years of observation for each person under observation at exact age x. Since no one is *added* to the study *at exact age x*, it should be clear that these individuals are those who are continued under observation from the prior interval. The next term, $(n/2)(_na_x - _nw_x - _nd_x)$, adds $n/2$ years of observation for each individual added to observation during the age interval x to $x + n$ under the assumption that additions are uniformly distributed during the interval and subtracts $n/2$ years of observation for each individual withdrawn alive or dying during the age interval x to $x + n$ under the assumption that withdrawals and deaths are uniform during the interval.

The next term, $(n/4)(_naw_x + _nad_x)$, may seem somewhat mysterious. Recall that $n/2$ years have been added for each addition during the period x to $x + n$ and that $n/2$ years have been subtracted for each withdrawal or death during the same period. The first two terms thus do not include any observation time for individuals added *and* withdrawn or added *and* dying in the same interval. The third term in Equation 8-4 counts $n/4$ years of observation for each such case. Why $n/4$? If additions are uniformly distributed, then on the average additions will come under observation halfway through the interval. If withdrawals and deaths are uniformly distributed, the additions who have come under observation halfway through the interval will leave halfway through the observation time remaining and thus will have been observed, on the average, for $n/4$ years. In other words, each such individual contributes $\frac{1}{4}$ of the length of the interval to the total observation time.

We now return to Table 8-3 and use it to calculate successive values of O_x. According to Table 8-3, there were no additions to observation before age 40 to

44; therefore there was no one under observation at *exact* age 40. Thus $O_{40} = 0$. A necessary first step is to identify an O_x value preceding the youngest age of observation so that we know it equals zero. We can then begin with this starting O_x value and, by adding $_na_x$ values and subtracting $_nw_x$ and $_nd_x$ values, derive subsequent O_x values:

$$O_{40} + {_5a_{40}} - {_5w_{40}} - {_5d_{40}} = O_{45}$$
$$0 + 1 - 0 - 0 = 1$$
$$O_{45} + {_5a_{45}} - {_5w_{45}} - {_5d_{45}} = O_{50}$$
$$1 + 2 - 0 - 1 = 2$$

By this process we derive all of the O_x values for our six-person example:

$$O_{40} = 0 \qquad O_{65} = 1$$
$$O_{45} = 1 \qquad O_{70} = 1$$
$$O_{50} = 2 \qquad O_{75} = 1$$
$$O_{55} = 1 \qquad O_{80} = 0$$
$$O_{60} = 2$$

Recalling that tallies in brackets in Table 8-3 represent deaths (all other observations that terminate are withdrawals) and that shaded cells represent additions and withdrawals or additions and deaths in the *same age interval*, we are ready to use Equation 8-4:

$$_5L_{40} = 5(0) + \frac{5}{2}(1 - 0 - 0) + \frac{5}{4}(0 + 0) = 2.50$$

$$_5L_{45} = 5(1) + \frac{5}{2}(2 - 0 - 1) + \frac{5}{4}(0 + 1) = 8.75$$

$$_5L_{50} = 5(2) + \frac{5}{2}(0 - 1 - 0) + \frac{5}{4}(0 + 0) = 7.50$$

$$_5L_{55} = 5(1) + \frac{5}{2}(2 - 1 - 0) + \frac{5}{4}(0 + 0) = 7.50$$

$$_5L_{60} = 5(2) + \frac{5}{2}(0 - 1 - 0) + \frac{5}{4}(0 + 0) = 7.50$$

$$_5L_{65} = 5(1) + \frac{5}{2}(1 - 1 - 0) + \frac{5}{4}(0 + 0) = 5.00$$

$$_5L_{70} = 5(1) + \frac{5}{2}(0 - 0 - 0) + \frac{5}{4}(0 + 0) = 5.00$$

$$_5L_{75} = 5(1) + \frac{5}{2}(0 - 0 - 1) + \frac{5}{4}(0 + 0) = 2.50$$

Since our detailed calculation of person-years of observation is summarized in ten-year age classes, we combine the five-year age class data into ten-year classes for comparison:

$$_5L_{45} + {_5L_{50}} = 8.75 + 7.50 = 16.25 = {_{10}L_{45}}$$

$$_5L_{55} + {_5L_{60}} = 7.50 + 7.50 = 15.00 = {_{10}L_{55}}$$

$$_5L_{65} + {_5L_{70}} = 5.00 + 5.00 = 10.00 = {_{10}L_{65}}$$

The values 16.25, 15.00, and 10.00 correspond to the exact values 12.56, 18.69, and 6.08, respectively, derived previously and shown in Table 8.2. For as few as six cases, there is no particular reason to expect a close match between the exact computation of person-years of observation and the formula computation, which assumes uniform distribution of additions, withdrawals, and deaths. For large bodies of data, however, the two methods usually agree quite well. Agreement can almost always be improved by summarizing data into narrower intervals of analysis.

By either method of calculating person-years of observation, the death rate per person-year of observation is obtained by dividing the number of deaths in specific age classes by the number of person-years of observation for that age class.

SAMPLING ERROR AND SIGNIFICANCE TESTS

As with all other types of statistics, person-year rates are subject to sampling error. Under the common assumption of uniform distribution of deaths within intervals of analysis, the standard error of a rate per person-year of observation can be estimated [83] as

$$\hat{SE}(_nm_x) = \left(\frac{_nm_x(2 - n\,_nm_x)}{_nL_x(2 + n\,_nm_x)} \right)^{1/2} \tag{8-5}$$

where

$_nm_x$ = rate per person-year for the age interval x to $x + n$
$_nL_x$ = number of person-years observed in the interval x to $x + n$
n = length of age interval

To illustrate the use of Equation 8-5, we return to the example of 36 cataract cases developing during 1300 person-years of observation, cited earlier in this chapter. The rate per person-year of .028 was for individuals age 69 to 71, and thus the length of the age interval is three years and $n = 3$:

$$\hat{SE}(_{71}m_{69}) = \left\{ \frac{.028[2 - (3)(.028)]}{1300[2 + (3)(.028)]} \right\}^{1/2} = .00445$$

and 95 percent confidence limits are .028 $\pm$ 1.96(.00445) = .019 and .037.

An alternative basis for estimating confidence limits for person-year rates is to assume the numerator of the rate to be a Poisson variable. If the rate is low (as it often is), this is not unreasonable. Recalling that for Poisson variables the square root of the parameter is the standard error of the statistic, we can define an upper limit to our 95 percent confidence interval as λ_U, where

$$\lambda_U = \text{observed number} + 1.96\sqrt{\lambda_U} \qquad (8\text{-}6)$$

Only 2.5 percent of all possible samples can be expected to result in an observed number smaller than $1.96\sqrt{\text{parameter}}$ below the parameter value. Thus, unless we happen to have a sample among this 2.5 percent, we can estimate the parameter value to be no greater than the observed number plus $1.96\sqrt{\text{parameter}}$, as in Equation 8-6.

Similarly, we can define a lower limit to our 95 percent confidence interval as λ_L, where

$$\lambda_L = \text{observed number} - 1.96\sqrt{\lambda_L} \qquad (8\text{-}7)$$

These equations are easy to solve if we recognize that Equation 8-6, for example, is a quadratic equation in $\sqrt{\lambda_U}$. In relation to the standard quadratic form $ax^2 + bx + c = 0$, $x = \sqrt{\lambda_U}$ and $x^2 = \lambda_U$. Putting Equation 8-6 into standard form and substituting 36, the observed number of cases from the cataract example, for c we have

$$\lambda_U - 1.96\sqrt{\lambda_U} - 36 = 0$$

then

$$\sqrt{\lambda_U} = \frac{-b \pm \sqrt{b^2 - 4ac}}{2a} = \frac{1.96 \pm \sqrt{3.84 - 4(1)(-36)}}{2(1)}$$
$$= 7.06 \text{ and } -5.10$$

Since the negative solution has no meaning in our problem, the solution is $\sqrt{\lambda_U} = 7.06$ and therefore $\lambda_U = 49.84$.

Following the same procedure for $\sqrt{\lambda_L}$, the equation to be solved is

$$\lambda_L + 1.96\sqrt{\lambda_L} - 36 = 0$$

and the solutions for $\sqrt{\lambda_L}$ turn out to be 5.10 and -7.06. Again the negative solution has no relevance so that $\sqrt{\lambda_L} = 5.10$ and $\lambda_L = 26.01$. (Because of the symmetry of the equations for $\sqrt{\lambda_U}$ and $\sqrt{\lambda_L}$, it is not necessary to solve both. In solving for $\sqrt{\lambda_U}$, we could have changed the sign of the negative solution and thus obtained the solution for $\sqrt{\lambda_L}$.)

By using the Poisson assumption, we have obtained 95 percent confidence limits of 26.01 and 49.84. Recalling that these are confidence limits on the numerator of the rate, i.e., the number of cataract cases occurring, we divide each of these by 1300 (considered not a sampling variable but a constant) to get 95 percent confidence limits on the person-year rate (via the Poisson approximation). These turn out to be .020 and .038, almost identical to the limits of .019 and .037 obtained with Equation 8-5. In both calculations, the presumption that $\pm$ 1.96 standard errors would yield 95 percent confidence limits depends on the distribution of all possible sample values being approximately normal. If the number of events is 20 or more (in our example it is 36), the normality assumption is probably satisfactory. To obtain more exact confidence limits for Poisson variables, see *Documenta* [84] and Bailar and Ederer [85] for methods and tables of values.

In Table 8-4, we recapitulate the assumptions underlying the calculation of person-year rates and compare them with the assumptions required for life table calculations. As can be noted from Table 8-4, if there are withdrawals, there are no differences of any practical importance. Since the methods for summarizing longitudinal observations by life table analysis or person-year analysis rest on the same assumptions, and since probability of risk is often numerically identical to rate of risk, does it make any difference which method is used? In my opinion there is no important distinction between the two methods and the choice between them need rest on nothing more than personal preference. My own preference is to use life table analysis when the cases observed have a common point for initiating observation (such as date of diagnosis or date of surgery) and where the dominant factor controlling risk is likely to be the time since that original date. For observation lacking this common initial date and where a major factor of risk tends to be age at observation, I prefer person-year methods.

Table 8-4. Assumptions Required for Summarizing Longitudinal Observations

Assumption	Life table method	Person-year method
1. Experience of persons after withdrawal (for any reason) is same as that of persons remaining under observation	x	x
2. Pooling relates to individuals with similar risk experience within interval of analysis	x	x
3. Withdrawals occur uniformly within interval of analysis	x	x
4. Constant risk within interval of analysis	x (only if there are any withdrawals)	x[a]

[a] Risks must be sufficiently low within intervals of analysis to permit k years of observation to reflect k times the risk of one year of observation.

NOTE

* To clarify the relationship between probability and rate, we consider identical populations at the start of an interval with no additions during the interval. The possibility of additions during the interval is not a serious problem for the person-year method, which uses average number at risk. For the life table method, however, additions during the interval are conceptually confusing at best. For this reason, one basis for choosing person-year analysis or life table analysis can be whether or not the data include additions to observation after the start of periods used for analysis. For more precise definitions of rate and risk see [82].

References

1. P. Armitage, *Statistical Methods in Medical Research*. New York: Wiley, 1971.
2. R. D. Remington and M. A. Schork, *Statistics with Applications to the Biological and Health Sciences*. Englewood Cliffs, N.J.: Prentice-Hall, 1970.
3. *J. Am. Stat. Assoc.* **47**:710 (1952).
4. The Rand Corporation, *A Million Random Digits*. Glencoe, Ill.: Free Press, 1954.
5. G. W. Snedecor and W. G. Cochran *Statistical Methods*, 6th edn. Ames: Iowa State University Press, 1967.
6. R. A. Fisher and F. Yates, *Statistical Tables for Biological, Agricultural and Medical Research*, Table XXXIII. London: Longman Group, 1974.
7. N. Mantel, *Am. Stat.* **23**:32 (1969).
8. A. M. Lilienfeld and D. E. Lilienfeld, *Foundations of Epidemiology*, 2nd edn. New York: Oxford University Press, 1980.
9. H. F. Dorn, *Hum. Biol.* **22**:238 (1950).
10. P. Pasquini, personal communication, 1980.
11. W. G. Madow and L. H. Madow, *Ann. Math. Stat.* **15**:1 (1944).
12. W. E. Deming, *Some Theory of Sampling*. New York: Wiley, 1950.
13. F. Ederer, *Am. J. Ophthalmol.* **79**:752 (1975).
14. M. Halperin, E. Rogot, J. Gurian, and F. Ederer, *J. Chron. Dis.* **21**:13 (1958).
15. J. L. Fleiss, *Statistical Methods for Rates and Proportions*, 2nd edn. New York: Wiley, 1981.
16. J. Cornfield, *J. Nat. Cancer Inst.* **11**:1269 (1951).
17. B. MacMahon and T. F. Pugh, *Epidemiology: Principles and Methods*. Boston: Little Brown, 1970.
18. J. S. Mausner and A. K. Bahn, *Epidemiology: An Introductory Text*. Philadelphia: Saunders, 1974.
19. J. H. Abramson, *Survey Methods in Community Medicine*, 2nd edn. Edinburgh: Churchill Livingston, 1979.
20. B. Woolf, *Ann. Hum. Genet.* **10**:251 (1955).
21. J. B. S. Haldane, *Ann. Hum. Genet.* **2**:309 (1956).

22. J. L. Fleiss, *J. Chron. Dis.* **32**:69 (1979).
23. N. Mantel, *Am. J. Epidemiol.* **106**:125 (1977).
24. O. Miettinen, *Am. J. Epidemiol.* **32**:80 (1979).
25. R. A. Hiller and H. A. Kahn, *Br. J. Ophthalmol.* **60**:283 (1976).
26. J. J. Gart, *Rev. Int. Stat.* **39**:148 (1971).
27. F. Ederer and N. Mantel, *Am. J. Epidemiol.* **100**:165 (1974).
28. D. Shurtleff, *The Framingham Study: An Epidemiologic Investigation of Cardiovascular Disease*, Section 26. Washington, D.C.: U.S. GPO, 1970.
29. J. Schlesselman, *Am. J. Epidemiol.* **99**:381 (1974).
30. J. Schlesselman, unpublished tables available from the author.
31. S. D. Walter, *Am. J. Epidemiol.* **105**:387 (1977).
32. M. L. Levin, *Acta Unio Int. Contra Cancrum* **9**:531 (1953).
33. J. Cornfield, W. Haenszel, E. C. Hammond, A. M. Lilienfeld, M. B. Shimkin, and E. L. Wynder, *J. Nat. Cancer Inst.* **22**:173 (1959).
34. S. D. Walter, *Biometrics* **32**:830 (1976).
35. P. Cole and B. MacMahon, *Br. J. Prev. Soc. Med.* **25**:242 (1971).
36. O. S. Miettinen, *Am. J. Epidemiol.* **99**:325 (1974).
37. S. D. Walter, *Int. J. Epidemiol.* **7**:175 (1978).
38. O. S. Miettinen, *Am. J. Epidemiol.* **91**:111 (1970).
39. L. Fisher and K. Patil, *Am. J. Epidemiol.* **100**:347 (1974).
40. U. S. Bureau of the Census, *Characteristics of the Population*, Volume 1, Part I, U.S. Summary Section I. Washington, D.C.: U.S. GPO, 1970.
41. National Center for Health Statistics, *Vital Statistics of the U.S.* Volume II, Part B. Washington, D.C.: U.S. GPO, 1970.
42. O. S. Miettinen, *Am. J. Epidemiol.* **100**:350 (1974).
43. L. L. Kupper and M. D. Hogan, *Am. J. Epidemiol.* **108**:447 (1978).
44. K. J. Rothman, *Am. J. Epidemiol.* **99**:385 (1974).
45. J. J. Schlesselman, *Case-Control Studies.* New York: Oxford University Press, 1982.
46. K. J. Rothman, *Am. J. Epidemiol.* **103**:506 (1976).
47. N. Mantel and W. Haenszel, *J. Nat. Cancer Inst.* **22**:719 (1959).
48. K. J. Rothman and J. D. Boice, *Epidemiologic Analysis with a Programmable Calculator*, NIH Publication 79–1649. Washington, D.C.: U.S. GPO, 1979.
49. O. Miettinen, *Am. J. Epidemiol.* **103**:226 (1976).
50. F. Yates, *J. Roy. Stat. Soc. Suppl.* **1**:217 (1934).
51. M. Halperin, Am. J. Epidemiol. **105**:496 (1977).
52. J. J. Gart, *Am. J. Epidemiol.* **115**:453 (1982).
53. O. Miettinen, *Biometrics* **25**:339 (1969).
54. N. R. Draper and H. Smith, *Applied Regression Analysis.* New York: Wiley, 1966.
55. M. S. Feldstein, *J. Roy. Stat. Soc.* **Series A**:61 (1966).
56. R. A. Fisher, *Ann. Eugenics* **7** (Part II):179 (1936).
57. J. Cornfield, T. Gordon, and W. W. Smith, *Bull. Int. Stat. Inst.* **38** (Part II):97 (1961).
58. J. Truett, J. Cornfield, and W. B. Kannel, *J. Chron. Dis.* **20**:511 (1967).
59. M. Halperin, W. C. Blackwelder, and J. I. Verter, *J. Chron. Dis.* **24**:125 (1971).
60. H. A. Kahn, J. B. Herman, J. H. Medalie, H. N. Neufeld, E. Riss, and U. Goldbourt, *J. Chron. Dis.* **23**:617 (1971).
61. A. A. Tsiatis, *Biometrika* **67**:250 (1980).
62. S. H. Walker and D. B. Duncan, *Biometrika* **54**:167 (1967).

63. D. G. Seigel and S. W. Greenhouse, *Am. J. Epidemiol.* **97**:324 (1973).
64. R. Prentice, *Biometrics* **32**:599 (1976).
65. T. R. Holford, C. White, and J. L. Kelsey, *Am. J. Epidemiol.* **107**:245 (1978).
66. Coronary Drug Project Research Group, *J. Chron. Dis.* **27**:267 (1974).
67. O. S. Miettinen, *Am. J. Epidemiol.* **104**:609 (1976).
68. A. C. Pigou, *Proc. Br. Acad.* **32**:13 (1947).
69. Diabetic Retinopathy Study Research Group, *Am. J. Ophthalmol.* **81**:383 (1976).
70. E. Rogot, *J. Chron. Dis.* **27**:189 (1974).
71. G. M. Matanoski, R. Seltser, P. E. Sartwell, E. L. Diamond, and E. A. Elliott, *Am. J. Epidemiol.* **101**:188 (1975).
72. L. M. Axtell, A. J. Asire, and M. H. Meyers, eds., *Cancer Patient Survival*, Report No. 5, HEW NIH Publication 77–992. Washington, D.C.: U.S. GPO, 1976.
73. C. L. Chiang, *Introduction to Stochastic Processes in Biostatistics*. New York: Wiley, 1968.
74. S. J. Cutler and F. Ederer, *J. Chron. Dis.* **8**:699 (1958).
75. C. L. Chiang in *Proceedings of the Fourth Berkeley Symposium on Mathematical Statistics and Probability* (J. Neyman, ed). Berkeley: University of California Press, 1961.
76. J. W. Kuzma, *Biometrics* **23**:51 (1967).
77. M. Greenwood, *Reports on Public Health and Medical Subjects* No. 33, Appendix 1. London: H. M. Stationery Office, 1926.
78. N. Mantel, *Cancer Chem. Rep.* **50**:163 (1966).
79. R. Peto, M. C. Pike, P. Armitage, N. E. Breslow, D. R. Cox, S. V. Howard, N. Mantel, K. McPherson, J. Peto, and P. G. Smith, *Br. J. Cancer* **35**:1 (1977).
80. National Center for Health Statistics, *Vital Statistics of the U.S.* Volume II, Section 5: Life Tables. Washington, D.C.: U.S. GPO, 1978.
81. H. S. Shryock and J. S. Siegel, *Methods and Materials of Demography* Volume 2. Washington, D.C.: U.S. GPO, 1975.
82. D. G. Kleinbaum, L. L. Kupper, and H. Morgenstern, *Epidemiologic Research*, Belmont, Calif.: Lifetime Learning Publications, 1982.
83. C. L. Chiang in *Vital Statistics, Special Report 47* (no. 9). Washington, D.C.: U.S. GPO, 1961.
84. *Documenta Geigy Scientific Tables*, 7th edn. Basle: Ciba-Geigy, 1970.
85. J. C. Bailar and F. Ederer, *Biometrics* **20**:639 (1964).

Index